Best Friends

the story of Dogs for the Disabled

by Sarah Carr and Jackie Williamson

Acorns Publishing

Published in 2009
by Acorns Publishing

A catalogue record for this book is available from the British Library

ISBN 978-0-9557375-6-5
Design, cover and typesetting by Elaine Sharples

Printed and bound in Great Britain by
CPI Antony Rowe, Chippenham and Eastbourne

Acorns Publishing
Pembrokeshire

www.acornspublishing.co.uk
email: acorns@acornspublishing.co.uk

Dedication

This book is dedicated to Jade, my little ray of sunshine and inspiration for writing this book, and to Jackie Williamson for believing in me.

Sarah Carr

Acknowledgements

I would like to thank all the people who have been involved and supported me during the years of writing this book.

Thanks must go to George Newns and Deborah Hay for their generous encouragement and their help with some of the facts about Frances. Also thanks to Doreen Cross, Neil Ewart and Helen McCain for information about the charity's early years. I am grateful to Daphne Townsend for contacting the family of Gladys Rainbow and for their generosity in providing me with a photo of the first partnership to qualify. I would also like to pay tribute to the late Colin Plum – founder of Dogs for the Disabled's Warwickshire Supporters' Group – for his constant support and encouragement of this and many other projects.

I am thankful to the Lyon family for lending me their computer so I could start to type the manuscript. I am also grateful to Peter Purves for the foreword and to Jillie Wheeler for allowing me to use her poem 'My Dog'.

Thanks too, to all the clients – and their dogs – for giving permission for their stories to appear in the book, to Fred and Jean Nicholls for sharing their experiences of puppy socialising and to Corrine Mitchell for her fascinating insight into what life can be like for a retired dog.

I am indebted to the chief executive of Dogs for the Disabled, Peter Gorbing, for his unwavering support and for writing chapter nine. I would also like to express my gratitude to all the trustees and staff of Dogs for the Disabled.

Jackie Williamson deserves a special mention. Without her
dedication, encouragement, excellent editorial skills and her
belief in me, 'Best Friends' would never have got into print.
Thanks also to my long suffering husband Martin and
Jackie's husband Mike for their patience during this lengthy
project.

I close with a final mention of Zach and Jade. Thanks for
the inspiration and the special times we shared.

Sarah Carr July 2009

'A dog believes you are what you think you are.'
(Jane Swan)

'We are alone, absolutely alone on this chance planet; and,
amid all the forms of life that surround us, not one,
excepting the dog, has made an alliance with us.'
(Maurice Maeterlinck – 'My Dog')

Dogs for the Disabled's Mission Statement

Creating Partnerships – Changing Lives

To train assistance dogs to provide practical support to disabled adults and children, and to provide disabled people and their families who have a dog with practical advice and support.

Contents

Foreword

One day, quite out of the blue, I received a letter from a young woman called Sarah Carr. She wanted to know if I would cut the ribbon on a charity walk she was helping to organise for Dogs for the Disabled. Little did I know, when I agreed to perform this small task, that it would be merely the start of an enduring, and rewarding, relationship with this charity that does so much to enrich the lives of disabled people.

The walk was a great success and was soon followed by another request – to be interviewed for Dogs for the Disabled's magazine. Next I was asked to present certificates to people who had recently qualified with their dogs, when I was given the great honour of being made a vice-patron of the charity. Then, before I knew it, the tireless Sarah Carr had written a book and was asking me to write the foreword!

Disability isn't just something that happens to somebody else. It isn't just something that some people are unlucky enough to be born with. And it isn't something that the rest of us should be turning away from, whether it's from our own embarrassment or as a way of pretending it isn't happening. Who knows what may be just around the corner for us?

Disability is something that can touch all our lives, as I

know too well. A few years ago I fell from the roof of my house when I was pruning some Virginia creeper and broke bones in both of my feet. With both legs encased in plaster, I was stuck in a wheelchair for nearly four months. It was a nightmare I thought I'd never wake up from. I'd gone, overnight, from being active and independent to someone who had to rely on help to do the simplest thing. But I was lucky. However bad it was for me, I knew it wouldn't last. I didn't have to face the knowledge that I would never recover and I will never know what it is like to be inside the soul of someone who is in that position.

Dogs for the Disabled was the first charity of its kind in the United Kingdom. It trains dogs to live and work in partnership with disabled people. These impressive animals carry out simple, every day tasks that their owners find difficult or impossible to do for themselves. But they do more than that. They also give disabled people back their independence, their confidence, their self respect and their will to go on. To find out how they do it, how it all came about and what the future holds for assistance dogs everywhere, read Sarah's personal account in the pages of this excellent book.

I am proud to be associated with Dogs for the Disabled and I wish the charity, its clients and, above all, its dogs a successful future.

Peter Purves
Vice-patron
Dogs for the Disabled

Chapter one

Perfect partners

Picture the scene. You're disabled, at home on your own in your wheelchair, getting ready to go out. Then you drop your keys. With a huge amount of effort, no little pain and at considerable risk of toppling over, you manage to pick them up. You wheel yourself to the door, struggle to get it open, manoeuvre yourself through and eventually manage to pull it shut behind you.

Or you could be ill in bed, with only the television for company. Bored with what's on you reach for the remote controller, drop it on the floor and it bounces away out of reach. You're doomed to watch the same channel, perhaps for hours, until someone comes home and helps you out.

Picture the scene again. This time help is at hand, in the shape of a trained assistance dog. No matter how many times you ask, he or she will willingly pick up your keys, open and close the door, bring you the remote or carry out a score of other tasks, whether you're at home, at work, out shopping or socialising. No pained expressions, no heavy sighs. Just a wagging tail, a desire to please and a huge zest for life.

Ask disabled people with assistance dogs what is so special about their particular dog, and the answers will always be the same. 'He's given me back my independence,' they will tell you. 'And freedom. And self respect'. Even though each dog is trained to suit the specific needs of just one person, they all bring to their owners these matching – and priceless – gifts.

Take Dick Thomsett, for example. As a young man Dick was a member of the original SAS. A real-life action man, he prided himself on his strength and fitness. These days, though, the elderly war veteran is more like the bionic man, with a metal plate in his hip and a tungsten thigh. Cataracts left him blind in one eye and with only half his sight in the other and to top it all he wears a hearing aid. He was lonely, isolated and virtually housebound. One day he fell over in his Northampton bungalow and it took him an hour to crawl to the emergency cord to call for help.

Then he got Pippa, a sleek black Labrador with silken ears, liquorice eyes and a turbo-driven wag to her tail. But she's more than just a beauty. Dick's life may one day depend on Pippa and her training – the next time he falls he knows that Pippa will immediately pull the cord for him, and raise the alarm in seconds.

Dick describes Pippa as his dream come true. She picks things up for him, pulls his socks off for him and barks for help if he asks her to. Even more than this, she gives him companionship, friendship and a purpose in life.

'We are a wonderful partnership, like butter to bread,' he says. 'One day when we were out shopping I looked round, and there was Pippa with my wallet in her mouth. I hadn't even noticed I'd dropped it, but she had. She picked it up for me and looked after it until I needed it.

'The quality of my life has so radically improved since I got Pippa and now I can't imagine what it was like before. I am very privileged to have such a wonderful, adorable dog. I don't have the words to describe what she means to me. She brings me so much happiness and joy and I hope I return it to her'.

Young Jamie Sutherland is more than fifty years younger than Dick, but he is just as devoted to his assistance dog as Dick is to Pippa. When Jamie was 14, he was involved in a road accident. He spent a year in hospital recovering from acquired brain injury and when he finally returned home it was in a wheelchair. Life became frustrating for the teenager. He found it difficult to do the simplest things for himself and he'd lost touch with most of his friends. Like Dick, Jamie felt isolated and lonely.

Three years after the accident Jamie's family heard about Dogs for the Disabled and he was introduced to a young yellow Labrador, Kandy.

'It was love at first sight,' says Jamie. 'Kandy came straight up to me and put her paws on the side of my wheelchair. I couldn't believe this beautiful dog was going to be mine. Until I got her I had lost the will to live. But now, because of her, people no longer see the wheelchair. They want to talk to me.'

To start with Kandy helped Jamie around the house but the pair's biggest challenge came when Jamie went to college.

'It was my first time living away from home and I'm not sure how I would have coped without Kandy,' Jamie recalls. 'But as soon as we got there everyone wanted to meet her and we soon had friends all over the campus. Without Kandy I would have felt different and isolated. The fact that she can help me with practical tasks as well as give me companionship is a key part of our relationship.'

Jamie's mother, Sharon, puts it more simply.

'Kandy gave Jamie a reason to live. She saved his life.'

Jamie and Kandy's partnership lasted until Kandy reached retirement age. She still lives with the family as a pet, and Jamie, now aged 29, has a new assistance dog, Tyler, a black Labrador.

Some people are born with a disability but for many more it is something that happens out of the blue, such as Jamie's, or gradually, like Dick's. That's how it was for Diane Dodge. Married with two grown-up daughters she enjoyed her part-time job as a bank clerk and her voluntary role as a guide dog puppy-walker. Diane was busy and active, never happier than when she was tramping across the fields near her Warwickshire home with her dogs. In 1987 everything changed. Diane was diagnosed with multiple sclerosis.

Over the next few years she gradually lost the use of her legs and right arm. The only way she could get around was in her electric wheelchair and she became increasingly dependent on other people. She mourned the loss of her self-reliance. She was used to doing things for herself and it was hard to keep asking for help.

'The hidden symptoms, such as the tiredness, were the

hardest to bear,' says Diane. 'I felt I needed a label pinned to me, saying 'I'm not lazy, I've got MS.'

Then she heard about Dogs for the Disabled and was introduced to Jago, a strikingly handsome golden retriever. The pair hit it off straight away and Jago soon learned to do the tasks that would give Diane back some of her independence.

Diane had to be trained too, as all Dogs for the Disabled clients are, to show she was able to look after Jago properly. It was a responsibility she did not take lightly.

'My main worry was that I wouldn't be able to live up to him, to do him justice. Such a lot of work had gone into training him and it would have been heartbreaking if I did something wrong and he had to go back'.

But she needn't have worried. She and Jago became great partners. When she asks him to do something he does it eagerly and happily, deep amber tail wagging and a big grin on his soft mouth.

Ask Diane what Jago does that makes such a difference to her life and she says it's the simple, everyday things that she used to take for granted.

'Yes, I can struggle to close the door, but he does it easily. He helps empty the washing machine and tumble drier, and he fetches the phone for me. If I'm upstairs and need something from downstairs, he'll go and get it. He picks things up when I drop them – today it was my lipstick. If I didn't have Jago I would have had to leave my lipstick on the floor until my carer came. It's things such as these that make life easier, the little things that mean so much. It's the companionship and the extra security of knowing he's there for me. He's my best friend.'

Jago, of course, has an ulterior motive. He knows that being a good boy and helping Diane usually – but not always – results in a treat. Assistance dogs are trained on the principle of rewards for good behaviour, but they are not rewarded every time. It's like playing a fruit machine. Sometimes you win, sometimes you don't, but it's the expectation of a win that keeps you playing. It's the same with dogs. They never know when they will get a reward but they're always hoping.

Jago worked this out a long time ago, and came up with a way of rewarding himself.

'When I ask him to do something he puts his toy in my lap first, does the task then comes back for his toy,' Diane explained. 'And the great thing is, you can't be depressed when you've got a dog around. Especially one as clever as Jago.'

But Jago isn't the only clever assistance dog. Tim Hockin's Olivia even taught herself how to fold things up! Tim wears a kilt because it's cool, comfortable and convenient, so in the winter he wears long socks to keep warm. When Olivia takes off his shoes and socks at night she naturally 'folds them up' by picking them up in the middle! Of course, the humans always respond by making lots of fuss of her and this spurs her on to even cleverer things. What she really finds fun is pulling off Tim's one-metre lengths of elastic bandage. She has to go a long way backwards, because they stretch, and then they twang up past her nose. They also get picked up in the middle and neatly folded by Olivia. More rewards follow.

Olivia has what are known as 'neat teeth' which means she can crunch a single Rice Krispie. This, of course, never fails to produce cries of 'Oh, how clever – how does she do it?' together with lots of pats, cuddles and rubs of the tickly spot towards the back of her tail. Olivia gives the clear impression that she thinks humans are very easily entertained.

Olivia is a yellow Labrador retriever cross who was originally trained to be a guide dog but, unfortunately, could not be relied upon not to chase cats. Tim says this inclination is still evident but is overcome when she is out with him by the fact that he and his electric powered wheelchair together weigh approximately 250 kilograms – and Olivia is firmly attached by a strong leather lead. The happy result of her unfortunate habit is that she was passed on to Dogs for the Disabled and retrained to help in ways other than guiding. Tim says he is extremely glad God gave Olivia a cat-attraction complex because otherwise he wouldn't have had the most wonderful companion a person could want.

'People always ask what does she do to help me and I find it very difficult to explain that it isn't just that she does so many things for me, but the way in which she does them. It's her attitude, the fact that she so obviously enjoys doing them. Even a simple request to find a dropped handkerchief is the start of a fun couple of minutes for both of us.

'Yes of course she undoes my shoe laces for me when I'm

going to bed, passes me my shoes when I get them off and takes my socks off for me. Yes, she helps with pullovers, jackets or shirts. Yes, and fetches the phone from wherever I've left it, picks up the door key when I drop it and picks up anything else that I drop for that matter. And of course she will speak when I ask her to, to get someone to come and help me when I need it, go backwards, forwards, left or right, sit, stand, stay, go on, come back or just about anything I ask her.

'But it's not just the ordinary things she does that make her special. It's the way she makes a big fuss of me when the MS is being more of a bummer than usual, and the fact that I can tell her how fed up I am without getting a "buck yourself up" reply. And she never says she knows how I must feel!'

One night while Tim was still able – just – to get into bed by himself, he was alone at home in Hampshire while his wife Nadine was visiting her mother. Things started to go wrong in the bathroom and Tim ended up lying across the foot-rests of his wheelchair, jammed against the door. On the other side of the door were Olivia and the cordless phone. His mobile phone was in the bag on his wheelchair, in easy reach for Tim when he was sitting in the chair but three inches out of his reach when he was lying on the foot-rests. Those three inches may as well have been three miles.

On the other side of the door, Olivia was clearly distressed at not being able to help her master. It took Tim seventy five long and painful minutes to get the door open six inches. Olivia took the phone to him and he rang for help. Tim insists there was nothing particularly special about this. Every assistance dog owner could tell a similar story, he says.

But it was what the ambulance crew found when they arrived that makes Olivia's intelligence and loyalty really stand out. Outside the bathroom door were three TV remote controllers and a pullover, all neatly laid out. Olivia was so worried at hearing Tim's struggles that she'd brought everything she could think of that might help.

'Special?' says Tim. 'You have to believe it!'

Most Dogs for the Disabled clients will tell you about the reassurance they get from having a specially trained assistance dog around. Wendy Morrell even sleeps better at night, knowing her dog Caesar is there to look after her.

A short conversation with Wendy quickly reveals an intelligent woman who refuses to let her disability get in the way of what she wants to do. Since being partnered with Caesar in 2000 she finds her life is busier than she ever imagined it could be and she is getting more adventurous by the day. With her handsome four-footed escort by her side Wendy has the confidence to travel by train, boat and aeroplane again and Caesar, a golden retriever, is the first assistance dog to have accompanied his owner to Wimbledon.

Disabled in her teens, Wendy nevertheless maintained a full and active life but a sporting accident in 1989 resulted in brain damage. As a result she has dizzy spells and problems with her memory. It is the most ordinary things that Caesar does that make him extraordinary to Wendy. Her memory problems mean that she sometimes forgets where she has left things and she remembers one incident before she had Caesar when she searched for more than four hours for some keys. She was in tears by the time a carer came and realised she had left them in a pair of trousers earlier in the day. She couldn't even remember changing out of them.

Things are very different these days. Caesar won't let her leave the house without her keys and if she gives the instruction 'find keys' he searches all the usual places until he tracks them down.

Wendy says before she had Caesar her anxiety levels were always very high. 'I used to get frustrated at the slightest thing or go into a downward spiral of depression because I dropped something and couldn't pick it up. I used to sleep appallingly badly, listening out for the slightest noise, but I sleep very well now because I know Caesar would wake up and alert me if there was anything outside.'

Perhaps the best thing about Caesar is that, because of him, Wendy no longer falls out of bed – something that used to happen frequently. Wendy's brain damage means that she frequently drops items such as pens or paper. She used to lean out of bed to try and pick them up and, losing her balance, fall off the bed. This usually left her with bruises but, worse than that, it hurt her pride. These days Caesar happily picks things up for her and the undignified tumbles are all in the past.

'Caesar is everything I wanted and more,' she says. 'He is priceless because of what he does and the independence he gives me has improved my self esteem and given me back my identity. Before I got him friends asked if it was a good idea for me to have a dog and suggested he might tie me down. In reality his effect on my life has been the opposite. I now go out more and find myself getting involved with things that I would have been scared to do before. I have made new friends through the things I do with Caesar and he is an icebreaker when I'm out shopping or taking him for a walk.

'I got to the stage where I just couldn't be bothered to try anything new but now I never stop. I'm even teaching Caesar to help me with new tasks and it gives me a real lift when we're successful. He's just such a wonderful animal and he even has his own website, www.k9assistance.co.uk.

'It would be really difficult to recount briefly all the opportunites and experiences I have had since being partnered with Caesar, but some of the most memorable ones have taken place when we have been travelling together. We've dined in the members' dining room at the House of Commons in London, in the Senators' Dining Room on Capitol Hill, Washington DC, and more recently given a presentation together at European Pet Night at the European Parliament in Brussels. In 2008 I was really honoured to be accompanied by Caesar as we took part in the Olympic Torch Relay, carrying the Olympic torch across London Bridge. I have become involved with the assistance dog movement internationally, and now sit on various committees advising on aspects of life for people with disabilities and assistance dog partners in particular.

'With Caesar at my side, I have been able to rekindle my previous love of travel; he's probably one of the best travelled assistance dogs in the UK, and for all his dedication to work, I'd still say he's a dog who loves life. I wept tears of joy watching him when we went on a whale watching trip off San Diego in 2006: he was mesmerised by the sight of whales and dolphins alongside our boat. Even when they had gone he kept one eye on the horizon, looking out for whatever experience was to come next!'

Nicola Dunn, a lawyer from Birmingham, is also amazed at how many new tasks she has taught her assistance dog, Will, over the months. Nicola has been disabled all her life and until she got Will she had to rely on members of her family or other carers to do things for her. Now she says Will has turned her life around, giving her freedom and independence. And Nicola isn't the only one to have fallen for the charms of her beautiful golden retriever – her family all love him too, even though they weren't keen on dogs before he came into their lives.

'When I first met Will,' says Nicola, 'my initial thoughts were, "He's huge. I'll never be able to convince him to work in partnership with me". So I'm quite surprised at how much I have taught him over the months. Duncan Edwards, my instructor, taught me to have very high standards when training Will and not to accept anything less! It requires a lot of dedication and determination but it's great when he picks up a new task.'

Will helps Nicola by:
picking up things she has dropped
answering the telephone and bringing it to her wherever she

is in the house
fetching the mail in the morning
posting letters
operating lift buttons
searching for, and finding, named articles
pulling the duvet on and off Nicola's bed
putting washing in the machine
letting friends or carers in and out of the house
carrying documentation
speaking on request
opening and closing the doors to her office
fetching her slippers from upstairs or downstairs
taking items off shelves and placing them on the counter
when shopping
carrying shopping
putting rubbish in the bin
telling her when to get off at the right bus stop

So what does all this mean to Nicola? Let her tell you in her own words.

'Will gives me confidence and independence. I now no longer need to rely totally on carers to do even the simplest task. Before I had him I did not have the confidence to catch a bus into town and go shopping by myself. I will never be able to thank Dogs for the Disabled enough for giving me the opportunity to turn my life around. The charity also provides me with continuous help and support and, most important of all, it has given me my best friend!'

Such is the nature of illness and disability that

partnerships sometimes end not when the dog retires but
when its human partner dies. This is all the more poignant
when the dog has given hope and independence to someone
for whom there was little hope and no independence until
the dog's arrival. It was like that for John Wyatt, whose best
friend in the final months of his life was Freya, a small and
pretty, champagne coloured Labrador bitch. John had motor
neurone disease, a progressive condition for which there is
no cure. It affects the motor nerve cells, which relay signals
from the brain to the muscle groups, causing the neurones to
degenerate and leading to weakness and wasting of the
muscles. By the time he met Freya, John had already lost
the use of much of his upper body and the disease was
beginning to spread to his legs. It is largely thanks to
Professor Stephen Hawking, the respected scientist and
writer who also has motor neurone disease, that people in
the UK have become more aware of the illness and the havoc
it can wreak in the human body whilst leaving the intellect
intact.

It was one of John's carers who first sowed the seed about
having an assistance dog. John had never even had a pet dog
before but the idea interested him and he applied, all the
time wondering if he would be considered because of the
degenerative nature of his illness. However, after an
interview, the instructors at Dogs for the Disabled agreed
that a dog could help him.

All the assistance dogs trained by the charity have a
basic 'tool kit' of tasks, similar to the basic jobs that Pippa,
Kandy, Jago, Olivia, Caesar and Will carry out for their

owners. These everyday days jobs help their human partners to remain independent for as long as possible. But all the dogs are taught to do additional, specific things for their humans as well. In Freya's case it was to provide John with the comfort of knowing that if he fell she would bark for help.

From the moment they met, Freya was the light in John's life. She gave him confidence and security, as well as providing fun and becoming a trusted companion. A close friend, who watched him go through the last five years of his life, saw the difference in him after Freya arrived.

'The sparkle returned to his eyes. She gave him something to live for – a reason to carry on.'

Before John became ill he lived a normal life. He never had to ask people to help him and did not worry about what others were thinking. One of the horrors of motor neurone disease is its ability to strip sufferers of their independence. For John, being able to ask Freya to do some of the things he was no longer able to do for himself made a huge difference to his day-to-day life.

'Freya doesn't judge me, and when I feel down she is there for me,' he used to say.

In the short time John and Freya were together she changed his life. She gave him back the will to live.

Following John's death in December 2002 Freya was retrained and became the best friend of another disabled person.

Chapter two

The power of the dog – Sarah's story

Jade walked into my life and put a smile back on my face. Our first meeting was one I will never forget. The date was February 26, 1998 and the venue was the Assembly Rooms, Derby. Clients, staff and volunteers from the charity Dogs for the Disabled were out in force to support snooker star Steve Davis in his quest to win his first round match against Nigel Bond in the Liverpool Victoria Charity Challenge. In this contest snooker aces played for nominated charities over seven frames and Dogs for the Disabled was Steve's charity.

I took my seat in the front row. Looking across to my right I saw a black and white dog frantically making its way towards me with Dogs for the Disabled's training manager in hot pursuit. Moments earlier the dog had been startled by a bursting balloon and was clearly stressed. As soon as she reached me she sat down beside me and rested her head on my lap. From that moment on I couldn't take my eyes off her. I remember thinking 'you will do for me'.

In between watching Steve winning his frames, I found out more about the dog. Jade was a Border collie/golden retriever cross and she was the sponsorship dog for the event. Steve won the match and, more importantly, won enough money to sponsor Jade throughout her working life. A competition on Dogs for the Disabled's stand at the show invited visitors to name the sponsorship dog. Several themed names were put forward but the most popular, not surprisingly, was Snooks. Television presenter Anthea Turner, at that time patron of the Liverpool Victoria Charity Challenge, was on hand for the official naming ceremony and Jade revelled in her temporary new identity, not to mention all the attention that came with it. Shortly after this, Anthea became a vice-patron of Dogs for the Disabled.

Jade was born on November 14, 1995 to Kizzie, a Border collie brood bitch belonging to The Guide Dogs for the Blind Association. Kizzie cared for Jade and her other puppies for the first few weeks of their lives but Jade was destined to work for a living. At the tender age of six weeks, she made her first big move to live with her puppy walker, Janet Furber and her family, on the outskirts of Crewe.

Over the following twelve months Janet taught Jade all the social skills and basic obedience she needed as a future guide dog. Janet says she really enjoyed Jade's time with her. 'She was quite a character and always had such a glint in her eye – and of course she was a very attractive dog.'

Right from the start, Jade made a big impression on people wherever she went. She was the puppy walking Furber family's eleventh puppy and while they were caring for her, puppy number nine, Parker, returned to live with them permanently. Jade and Parker took to each other right away and were soon inseparable, curling up together to sleep and, of course, never passing up an opportunity to play. A favourite game involved Parker swimming in the canal near their home while Jade ran up and down the bank barking madly at him. Parker was good for Jade in other ways, too, and it was from mimicking his behaviour that she learned to come when she was called. The two young dogs became so close that when Jade left to start her training Parker pined for her and was quite unhappy for a while.

Jade's training began in earnest at The Guide Dogs for the Blind Association's centre in Bolton. She eventually qualified as a guide dog, but she never took to the work. I like to think she decided on a career change and applied for a job at Dogs for the Disabled, for which I will always be grateful.

Of course it wasn't quite like that! Jade had a very inquisitive mind and found what she considered to be the repetitive nature of guide dog work tedious. She never knew what I would ask her to do or when I would ask her to do it, so she was always alert for my next command. Assistance dogs have to have different characteristics from guide dogs, and she fitted the bill perfectly.

After she joined Dogs for the Disabled Jade's natural retrieving instincts came in very handy and she was quick and eager to learn new tasks. All she asked in return was that she got more cuddles and fuss than any other dog on the block, but that was easy. All she had to do was turn on the charm to melt the hearts of everyone around her.

A month after our first meeting Jade and I were together again, this time at Crufts, where we spent a day helping out on the Dogs for the Disabled stand. While she and I continued to get to know each other better, the charity's trainers were using the opportunity to see if we were a suitable match. This was a nerve-wracking time for me as I'd really set my heart on her but fortunately the trainers must have liked what they saw. A week later Linda Hams, the training manager at the time, brought Jade to visit me at home and at the end of the visit she told me what I'd been waiting all these weeks to hear. Jade and I were going to be an item. We could go forward and train together. I was delighted.

On April Fools' Day 1998 we began our training from home. I knew there would be a lot of hard work for us both as Jade was a natural leader and could be rather stubborn. It was a difficult first day for us as she had a stomach upset and I had to starve her for 24 hours – not an ideal way to start any relationship, let alone one as important as this.

The training sessions were long and tiring for dog, client and trainer but we progressed at a steady pace, despite the odd hiccup. As part of the course we had to take a night walk, which was designed to finish at a nearby hostelry. That night our walk took more than five hours to complete ... and we only went a mile each way. The problem was that Jade thought she was going for a free run and was convinced everything that moved was worth pulling for – even lamp posts become very interesting in the dark. Although dogs' night vision is better than ours they still rely more on air and wind scent in poor light, rather than sight. On the night in question, Jade repeatedly fixed her eyes on stationary objects some distance away, convinced they were about to move. She prepared to pounce on her prey if necessary, which made my task all the more difficult, particularly as my night vision is even poorer than the average human's. We arrived home very late, tired and hungry ... but at least we got our pint at the pub.

Five weeks later Helen McCain, our instructor at the time and now the charity's director of training and development, considered Jade and me safe enough to go out on the streets alone and Jade's blue training jacket was duly replaced with a yellow one to show the world she was now a qualified assistance dog. I signed a legally binding contract with Dogs for the Disabled, agreeing to adopt and look after Jade, and handed over my £1.00 qualification fee – such a small price to pay when you think what I was getting in return. The fee has since risen to £25, which is still the best value for money around. Each dog is given a registration number on qualification and Jade became the 150th dog to be successfully trained by Dogs for the Disabled, a real milestone in the charity's history.

Two days later we met Steve Davis again and I was able to thank him for his generosity in sponsoring Jade. It was a great occasion for me and a happy reunion for Jade and her famous sponsor.

We had our photographs taken together and gave interviews to Mad about Dogs magazine and local newspapers, before taking our seats to watch Steve play Ronnie O' Sullivan in an exhibition match. Steve is a charming person and told the assembled audience, 'These well trained dogs make a real difference to the quality of life of a disabled person. I am delighted to have met Sarah and seen Jade in action and contributed to the Charity's 150th qualification.'

I found him friendly, easy to talk to and genuinely interested in hearing about Jade's progress. I told him what a difference Jade had made to my life and how much more confident I was since getting her. She was my little ray of sunshine. Only that afternoon she had saved me from a very muddy situation. She was enjoying a free run when I got stuck in mud on my mobility scooter and started to sink. I blew my whistle twice and Jade returned to my side. I asked her to sit and to speak. To my relief she did bark, and kept barking until help arrived and I was rescued. This may not seem significant but Jade was only taught to bark on command a week before I had her. When she was a guide dog her barking skills were not required but I needed her to alert attention if necessary. Although this incident happened scarcely three weeks after we started training together, Jade instinctively knew there was something wrong. I was very proud of her and I realised then a strong bond had already developed between us.

Jade and I continued to be monitored by Dogs for the Disabled's training department and as our confidence grew so did our teamwork skills. Training didn't just end for us both the day we qualified and part of the ongoing monitoring process looked at ways of developing Jade's skills to suit my particular needs. She rapidly became efficient and competent in a wide range of tasks including emptying the washing machine and fetching the post and newspapers from the doormat. This might not sound particularly spectacular but it made a world of difference to me as I have arthritis and fibromyalgia. This is a condition in which the muscles and tendons around the joints start to swell and a burning pain ensues. The condition affects many parts of the body and during a flare-up the tender points become excruciatingly painful, even to the slightest touch. Chronic fatigue and sleep disturbance is also a big problem with this illness. It is an unpredictable condition with recurrent attacks lasting from a few hours to many months.

Before Jade came along I would have to leave simple domestic routines to my husband, Martin, which was frustrating for me and tedious for him. It is only when you have to keep asking other people to do things for you that you really appreciate what it means to be able to do them for yourself. Having Jade meant I was now independent for the first time since my illness struck, ten years previously.

Outside the confines of the house I taught Jade to take the washing from the laundry basket and give it to me to hang on the line. This was when I discovered what a quick learner she is. I pegged out the first item she gave me and turned round to ask her to get the next one. I needn't have bothered. She was already sitting there with a towel hanging from her mouth and her expression clearly saying, 'What took you so long?'

Jade was a sensitive dog and needed a lot of persuasion to pick up my crutches and close the door behind us when we left a room, jobs that she seemed reluctant to do. She didn't like the feel of the cold metal crutches in her mouth and it worried her that the door was still coming towards her while she was going backwards, away from it. Instructor Chris Wilsdon, who by this time was helping with our training, came to the rescue and suggested I taped a big woolly sock around the handle of a crutch and then ask Jade to fetch the sock. Of course, when she picked up the sock she also picked up the crutch and earned lots of praise for getting it right. Chris and I decided to harness one of her natural instincts by encouraging her to close the door by tugging on a rope when asked to 'pull'. That way she overcame her dislike of closing doors. We developed the technique to use 'pull' for taking off my coat and gloves, undoing shoelaces and removing footwear. This just goes to show that with a bit of imagination, some lateral thinking and lots of love, nothing is impossible.

Jade shared my energetic personality and as soon as I picked up the keys for my electric scooter Jade was there, ready and eager to be off. She would trot beside the scooter, wagging her tail and getting more and more excited the nearer we got to the post office. Once there, she knew exactly what to do. Taking my allowance book gently in her mouth she would jump up, placing her front paws on the counter.

Once the postmaster had taken the book from her she would sit next to me and wait to be called again, perhaps several times. The final time was always special for Jade, as she knew the postmaster kept a treat behind the counter for her. This was such a familiar part of her routine that she wouldn't leave the post office without it.

A long queue of customers would always develop behind me, with everyone marvelling at Jade and what she'd been doing. Before Jade came along, shopping used to take twenty minutes but with my assistance dog everyone stopped to say hello to her and I had to allow at least an hour.

But life for Jade wasn't all work. We had a lot of fun together and she really was one of the family. She got on well with our three cats and even thought of herself as an honorary feline. One day I came down to breakfast to find a mass of feathers and a terrified sparrow hiding under the sideboard. Martin carefully moved the cats' breakfast delicacy out of harm's way into the front garden, but the bird obviously had suicidal tendencies and made its way back towards the house. When I opened the garage door it hopped in and took cover under a table, tweeting furiously. By this time the cats had completely lost interest, but Jade hadn't: she spent the next twenty minutes trying to get the sparrow out again. Her paws-off approach eventually met with success and it flew off, unharmed, its faith in big black 'cats' thoroughly restored!

I had first contacted Dogs for the Disabled in March 1994. I studied the criteria for applying for an assistance dog and realised that I qualified. After careful consideration, I completed the application form and Dogs for the Disabled obtained medical reports to make sure that having an assistance dog would not harm my health any further. Once the trainers were satisfied with the reports they visited me at home to discuss my needs and asked me to think about the ways in which a dog could help. At that time, my biggest need was for a dog to help me with my balance when walking and standing.

My name was put on the waiting list and the charity told me I would go for training once they found me a suitable dog. I knew it was unlikely to happen overnight as the trainers and instructors are very careful about getting just the right match between dog and client and this often takes time. I played the waiting game for three years. Two potential suitors visited me in that time but, for one reason or another neither was an ideal match.

In February 1997, I spent a day at Dogs for the Disabled's head office at Ryton-on-Dunsmore, to 'work out' with a couple of dogs. Zach, a black Labrador, came bounding into the training room. Chris Wilsdon, Zach's trainer, demonstrated some basic obedience moves. Then it was my turn. I am sure Zach and I were as nervous as each other. My head was spinning with commands – sit, down, wait, stay … or should that be sit, wait, down, stay? All this, and I had to keep my eye on the dog, demonstrate good voice control and look where I was going, all at the same time. Before we started the exercise I thought, 'Oh help!' Then I looked into the dog's intelligent brown eyes and put my trust in him. Amazingly, he did respond to my voice although, naturally, he did look to Chris for reassurance. Chris and Zach left the room and Helen entered with Gabby, a golden retriever . Helen demonstrated some simple retrieval exercises. I had a go, but found that the dog was not responding to me.

I returned home and was asked to take Zach for a short

walk, with him trotting beside my scooter. That completed the day's training. Helen then asked me if I would like to go forward to train with Zach! My dream had finally come true.

We started a two-week training course at Wokingham Guide Dog Centre in March 1997 but I returned home after four days because Gabby and Zach went down with kennel cough. We eventually continued our training at the Ryton-on-Dunsmore centre and qualified a few weeks later.

Zach was another example of a dog that originally started his training with The Guide Dogs for the Blind Association. In his case the trainers found he was too easily distracted from guiding so Guide Dogs donated him to Dogs for the Disabled. Unfortunately, a short time after our qualifying period, he showed signs of 'switching off' whenever I asked him to do anything, particularly emptying the washing machine. Perhaps he didn't approve of my brand of washing powder. Whatever the reason, he absolutely refused to retrieve the clean washing although he was happy enough to take out his dirty old tea towel that we used for training. Ten months into my partnership with Zach, when he was four years old, Dogs for the Disabled decided to retire him on health grounds. He returned to the Gibson family, his puppy walkers in Yorkshire where, to this day, he runs in green fields to his heart's content. According to Mr Gibson, Zach continues to enjoy his retirement to the full. His favourite pastime is chasing hares but of course, he never catches them and if he did he wouldn't know what to do with them. I guess it's just a dog's life!

Chapter three
In the beginning ...

Born on August 19, 1949 Frances Marylyn Newns grew up in India, Singapore and Australia. She had many interests but her main passions were athletics, horses and dogs.

She was diagnosed with bone cancer when she was just fifteen and flew to England from Australia to have a half thigh amputation on her left leg. This type of amputation usually makes it more difficult to use an artificial limb because of the absence of the knee joint. But Frances was successfully fitted with a prosthesis and resumed a near normal life. She later married Jim Hay and they made their home in Bellemere Road, Hampton-In-Arden. Their daughter, Deborah was born on August 23, 1977. The family broke up a few years later and Frances and Deborah eventually moved to Brook House, Lower Ladyes Hills, Kenilworth.

Frances always had pet dogs and enjoyed training them to perform tricks and tasks, something for which she had a natural talent. This early close affinity with dogs proved invaluable when Kim, her Belgian Shepherd bitch, showed the bond between them could go far beyond that of a human and a pet dog – she seemed instinctively to know when Frances needed help to get out of chairs or climb the stairs.

Frances quickly realised the potential of training a dog to help disabled people and with this idea firmly fixed in her mind, Dogs for the Disabled was born in October 1986. The next step was to recruit like-minded people. Over the next two years Frances had to overcome many hurdles before Dogs for the Disabled became a formally registered charity. She began a tireless campaign of interviews and talks, as well as promoting her charity on local and national radio, television and newspapers.

Her first project was to find a dog as a companion for the residents of a local retirement home. She scoured the region's dog rescue centres and met more than seven hundred dogs before making her choice. Holly was a terrier cross who turned out to be a big hit with residents and staff at the home in Kenilworth.

Frances' delight in handing Holly over in December 1986 was twofold. Not only had an unwanted dog been given a fine new home but she also brought happiness to nine elderly people, in the form of four legs and a wagging tail.

In the early days Frances set up an advisory management committee, one of whose members was Ian Burr, a solicitor. He drew up a draft Declaration of Trust, which formed the basis for the constitution and was approved by the Charity Commission. Dogs for the Disabled became registered charity number 700454 on June 27,1988 with Frances as director general. Brook House was the headquarters; the members of the management committee became trustees and for the next two years they took it in turns to chair the monthly meetings. This rotating chair system changed in 1989 when Dick Lane, FRAgS, FRCVS became chairman, a role he undertook until 1995 and again from 1997 until early 2003, when he retired.

The benefits of owning a dog are well documented. Disabled people feel more part of the community when people speak to their dog and at the same time passers-by marvel at the union of dog and disabled person. Having a dog gives disabled people the confidence to speak to others and helps rescue them from their social isolation: when you have a dog, people speak to you on equal terms.

Research surveys among clients of Dogs for the Disabled, carried out in 1995 and again in 2000 by June McNicholas and a team from the Department of Psychology at the University of Warwick, proved the value of assistance dogs to disabled people. Not only can the dogs be trained to help disabled people with a range of valuable practical tasks, the surveys found, but 'they also contribute significantly to their owners' social, psychological and physical well-being'.

June McNicholas was a friend of Frances Hay and her team has a worldwide reputation for its work in examining the relationships between animals and humans and the benefits they bring. Her research team found that Dogs for the Disabled clients enjoyed improved health and well-being, increased social contact and social and emotional support from the dogs. 'We found no client who regretted the decision to have an assistance dog and the vast majority (of those surveyed) expressed total satisfaction with the very positive changes that had come about after having an assistance dog.'

Zane was a moving example of this. The yellow Labrador was partnered with Rose Freeman after a stroke left her so disabled that she was unable to speak and had slight use in only one hand. Because she was unable to use her voice to tell Zane what she wanted him to do, Dogs for the Disabled trained him to respond to hand signals. The effect on Rose was dramatic. She was so overwhelmed by her wonderful dog and the difference he made to her life that she decided to have speech therapy so that she could speak to him.

Frances was adamant that rescue dogs should lead fulfilling lives and she made it her policy, where possible, to choose dogs that were unwanted, lost, or abandoned. She often quoted from Roger Caras' book A Celebration of Dogs: 'A dog is utterly sincere, it cannot pretend, it cannot act in any way patronising no matter how physically or emotionally incapacitated the human participant is.' Frances remained convinced that dogs have a natural affinity with people who are disabled, and act accordingly. They want to do the work, to help and to please: they are not forced into anything.

Tragedy struck early in 1987 when Kim, then aged about twelve, died from cancer of the spleen. Frances was devastated but she was all the more determined to make the charity succeed. On her travels around rescue centres she found Misty, a Siberian husky crossbreed who was found on the streets of Birmingham, close to death. Misty was a very affectionate dog and Frances decided to keep her as a companion. She often took Misty to talks and presentations, when she explained the benefits of owning a companion dog.

Later that spring, after an exhaustive search of rescue centres Frances, accompanied by her daughter Deborah and Jenny Cotton, a veterinary assistant, chose Rani to be trained as the first assistance dog. Jenny took Rani home and encouraged her to switch lights on and off, open doors and pick up the cordless phone. Jenny also had to train Rani, a German Shepherd bitch, to work with a wheelchair. Her training was supported by Omega pet foods and she was the charity's first official dog to qualify.

August 24-29 of the same year was declared Dogs for the Disabled Week in Kenilworth. Frances' father wheeled her through the streets of Kenilworth to promote the occasion. Then on August 26, in a blaze of publicity, Rani was handed over to Mrs Gladys Rainbow, an amputee from Rugby. Gladys was no stranger to the world of dogs as she used to breed corgis herself. The official presentation by the town mayor, Councillor Bob Wooller, was held at the De Montfort Hotel in Kenilworth. Frances was ecstatic. All her hard work had finally paid off. This was a first for Dogs for the Disabled and the first assistance dog to be trained in the United Kingdom. There were similar schemes in America and Holland but she had been unaware of them until after she started Dogs for the Disabled.

Frances' work was publicised in the local media and this led to her being invited on to the Derek Jameson morning radio programme on BBC Radio Two. There was a huge response to the show from members of the public who, in a nation of dog lovers, were moved by what they had heard. Frances knew there were many more disabled people than there were deaf or blind. Although she never studied official statistics for registered disabled, deaf, hard of hearing, blind or partially sighted people in England she knew she could fill a gap in the market. She used to say, 'One day, I hope that an assistance dog will be available to everyone who can benefit from one'.

Official statistics for 1987, when Frances was establishing the charity, show that there were 1,455,627 registered disabled of whom 1,230,000 were physically disabled.

By 1999, using the definition of disability derived from the World Health Organisation as 'the inability due to impairment, to perform activities in typical and personally desired ways in society', it was estimated that more than eight and a half million people in Great Britain had a disability. [Grundy et al (1999) Disability in Great Britain (1)] The need for assistance dogs grows ever greater.

As news of Dogs for the Disabled spread, donations began to arrive. This was a great relief to Frances as she often dipped into her own limited resources to keep the charity afloat. Frances was also keen to get sponsorship to help with the cost of feeding the dogs so she approached Hill's Pet Nutrition. Hill's organised a fund-raising appeal to raise £50,000, by getting people to collect labels from their dried and tinned food. For every label returned to them, Hill's donated money to the charity. The company has continued to support the charity to this day.

In 1987 Frances enlisted the help of volunteers for administrative duties, and took on two paid employees.

Doreen Cross from Kenilworth became her secretary and Carolyn Fraser from Coventry was taken on as the charity's dog trainer. Carolyn had trained with The Guide Dogs for the Blind Association in Bolton for eight years before returning to the Midlands to work with dog clubs. Deborah, Fran's young daughter, was never far away and proved to be a tower of strength to her mum by exercising and feeding the dogs and accompanying Frances on talks.

Frances had a great sense of fun and a wicked sense of humour. In March 1988 she re-enacted the Lady Godiva ride through Coventry to keep a lunch appointment with the Lord Mayor of Coventry, Jeff White. There were, however, two notable differences from the original Lady Godiva. Firstly, Frances was fully clothed and secondly, the horse was led by a dog to show how well trained the charity's dogs were. The Lord Mayor had already donated money to the charity, on the condition that Frances took him to lunch. Frances responded the only way she knew how, by getting as much publicity for Dogs for the Disabled as she could before keeping the important appointment.

Despite publicity stunts such as this, the serious business of dog training continued. Amber – another young German Shepherd bitch – was donated to Frances by a couple who were unable to give enough time to the dog. Amber was nearly wild when she first arrived. She would not walk to heel or come when she was called. With patience, perseverance and a little direction, Amber overcame her fears and was pressing light switches, collecting the post and picking up the cordless phone in just five weeks. Frances and

Amber soon became inseparable and Frances was glad of the opportunity to use her as the charity's first demonstration dog.

Shortly afterwards, Fran was admitted to hospital for emergency treatment and she called on friends to look after Amber. Again, tragedy struck. Amber was playing off the lead and on the trail of a scent when she disappeared through a hole in the fence. The trail led her to the railway track and into the path of an oncoming train. Frances was left devastated once more. She didn't know how she would cope.

But then along came Amie, a golden retriever puppy who was donated by a breeder. She was given the name Amie by local school children who chose it because *amie* is French for friend. Frances kept Amie at home for several months and trained her to collect the post, fetch the phone and open and close doors. When she was old enough she accompanied Fran and Misty on presentations. On one occasion Amie handed out leaflets to the audience – she loved working for Fran even though she was a pet dog. Misty and Amie were inseparable. Although Amie worked and Misty sat back and watched, it was Misty who was top dog – what Misty did, Amie did too.

By 1990 Frances' health had deteriorated and she spent a lot of her time in bed. Helen McCain, a qualified trainer with Guide Dogs, joined Dogs for the Disabled on secondment at the beginning of the year and took on the training of three dogs. This took the pressure off Frances and allowed her to rest more.

In October Frances held a party at a local hotel to thank everyone who had helped her to get the charity started. It was to be her last public appearance. She died on December 22, 1990 aged just forty-one.

Frances saw ten dogs blossom into fully trained assistance dogs between 1986 and 1990. Her death left a huge gap, both in the charity and in the lives of her friends, and the next few months proved difficult. The five trustees continued to run the charity, but they struggled to maintain the high profile that Frances had worked so hard to achieve.

From its earliest days, Frances and her father, George Newns, were adamant that Dogs for the Disabled should remain a charity in its own right and that Frances should always be recognised for her pioneering work. This mnemonic is one of her mottos:

W U F F – Work With Understanding, Forgiveness and Friendship.

Chapter four
A dream comes true

Dogs for the Disabled had to find new premises when Brook
House was sold in 1991. Help was at hand in the form of a
Portakabin in the grounds of Edmondscote Manor, The Guide
Dogs for the Blind Association's training centre at Royal
Leamington Spa. Doreen Cross continued to work for the
charity as secretary to the trustees and Linda Crawley
worked as part time administration assistant. Debbie Parry
and her dog for the disabled, Elton, joined the team as public
relations officers. They attended many events up and down
the country from cheque presentations to dog shows,
promoting the charity wherever they went. Elton even won
the title 'Career Dog of the Year' in 1996.

As people became more aware of the charity the demand
for trained dogs also grew. It soon became apparent that
more suitable accommodation would need to be found.

The Guide Dogs for the Blind Association (GDBA) had
their breeding centre at Tollgate, just outside Leamington
Spa. In the grounds of the centre was a bungalow. As a
result of staff relocation the bungalow was empty and Guide
Dogs offered it to Dogs for the Disabled. This was ideal
because a large part of the training for an assistance dog
takes place in a home environment. The bungalow contained

all the fixtures, fittings and comforts of a normal home and any necessary office furniture was fitted in around them. As a fitting tribute to the founder of the charity, the trustees re-named the bungalow Frances Hay House.

A major change took place in 1995 when, following discussions with the Charity Commission, it was agreed with GDBA that all the members of the training staff at Dogs for the Disabled would leave the charity and become directly employed by GDBA. The two charities agreed that GDBA would train Dogs for the Disabled in return for an agreed contract fee for each dog that qualified. This would allow Dogs for the Disabled to focus on raising funds to support this work and so a new fundraising manager, Peter Gorbing, was appointed to assist the charity to develop its fundraising capacity. The training staff now employed by GDBA continued to work from Tollgate. As part of this change, the number of trustees was reduced to five and three of the trustees were appointed by The Guide Dogs for the Blind Association, thus ensuring close links between the two charities were maintained.

During 1995 the fund-raising department relocated to premises at the Grange Engineering works in Deppers Bridge, a village close to Leamington Spa, because of the lack of space at Frances Hay House. Fund-raising staff continued to work there until January 1997, when The Guide Dogs for the Blind Association bought The Old Vicarage Kennels at Ryton-on-Dunsmore near Coventry. The house was redesigned to be used as offices and training rooms, which were shared between the two charities. Dogs

for the Disabled staff were again all under the same roof.
There were enough kennels for twenty-six dogs in training.

The contract arrangement was examined in 1997 by
GDBA as part of a thorough review of the Association known
as Project 9. The outcome of Project 9 was a commitment by
GDBA to extend the range of the services that they offered
to blind and visually impaired people. As part of the review,
they decided not to extend their dog-related services to
people other than those who are blind and visually impaired
and, consequently, the Dogs for the Disabled unit did not sit
comfortably within the Association's future plans.

Following extensive discussions between trustees and
staff, it was decided that members of staff working for GDBA
on the Dogs for the Disabled contract would, if they wished,
be transferred to Dogs for the Disabled from January 1,
2000. The timing of the staff transfer neatly coincided with
the opening of Dogs for the Disabled's new training centre
near Banbury and in January 2000 there was a formal
separation between Dogs for the Disabled and The Guide
Dogs for the Blind Association. Despite this, the two
organisations have continued to work together and enjoy a
productive relationship.

During their time at The Old Vicarage, Dogs for the
Disabled began to look at ways of expanding for the future.
To do this successfully, the charity needed a national
training centre. This was what Frances Hay had always
dreamed of. With the approval of the board of trustees, Peter
Gorbing, who is now the chief executive, applied to the
National Lottery Charities Board for a capital grant. The

application process was long and complicated. The first priority was to find a suitable location and accommodation. Kathana Kennels, a cattery and dog boarding kennels which also boasted a large training hall, came onto the market.

These kennels were ideally situated near Banbury in north Oxfordshire, just off junction 11 of the M40 and close to the railway station. Banbury town centre, with its easy access for disabled people and dogs in training, was also close by. The presence of Shopmobility was also an attraction. A registered charity, the National Federation of Shopmobility UK was established in 1990 to provide a national network to help people with disabilities gain independence and equal opportunity. Through Shopmobility schemes disabled people can register and borrow electric and manual wheelchairs and scooters, sometimes free of charge, making it easier to get around the town independently. In 2001 the National Federation of Shopmobility UK joined forces with the Enham Trust, which supports disabled people, and the Royal Association for Disability and Rehabilitation (RADAR). The aim of the combined organisation is to serve, support and work on behalf of people with disabilities throughout the UK.

The site for Dogs for the Disabled had to be secure and away from any large residential areas so that noise from the dogs would not disturb neighbours. Kathana Kennels fitted the bill perfectly, coupled with the fact that its seven acres of land, some of them in neighbouring Northamptonshire, meant there was enough space to build offices and an accommodation block. The existing training hall and kennels were kept and modified, saving the charity money, and the big ridge-and-furrowed field was an extra bonus, giving the dogs lots of space to run and play.

Peter Gorbing prepared the relevant documents to support the bid, and submitted the application. The National Lottery Charities Board awarded a grant of £597,595 in 1998. The grant was the largest amount awarded to any animal related charity. Planning permission was granted in February 1999 and the site was purchased the following month. Work finally started in mid-May 1999.

While building work was going on, Dogs for the Disabled started to form links with local businesses and supporters in Banbury. In September Anthea Turner, who was a vice-patron of the charity, came to Banbury and had photographs taken with all the businesses that had helped so far. Meanwhile, some volunteers rang round local shops to see if they would be willing to donate items to furnish the new accommodation block. The Banbury Lions helped to organise the day and Anthea gave press and radio interviews. She also donned wellies and a hard hat for a tour of the site which, at the time, still resembled a mud bath. Despite this, Anthea said she was impressed with everything she saw and she was pleased to be supporting such a worthwhile project.

The new building had offices for administration and fundraising staff as well as a three-roomed accommodation block. This was probably the most significant thing about the centre as it means that clients and dogs are able to stay together, on site, while they are being trained. The kennel block has large, clean and airy kennels with individual outdoor runs, a grooming parlour and shower room. The dogs' meals are prepared in the kitchen, which also has washing machines and driers so the never ending supply of wet towels and muddy blankets can be kept fresh and clean. The training hall, a barn-sized building with a large, fenced run is close to the kennels and the whole site is linked by a series of paths so all areas are easily accessible, which is particularly important for clients.

The Frances Hay Centre opened its doors on January 24, 2000. Despite a few technological hiccups in the early days, there was a great sense of achievement and everyone shared the feeling that the move heralded a time of growth and consolidation for the charity.

Dogs for the Disabled also had a satellite centre in Exeter that served a substantial client base in the south west and this was moved to Weston-Super-Mare in 2005. The charity also located an instructor in Yorkshire in 2002 and six years later, in 2008, it opened its first northern regional training centre at the Nostell Estate Offices near Wakefield in West Yorkshire.

September 12, 2000 was another memorable day for Dogs for the Disabled. Despite a national petrol shortage, staff, supporters, clients and dogs gathered in the early autumn sunshine to see the Frances Hay Centre officially opened by Deborah Hay, the founder's daughter. Tom, a young black Labrador in training, pulled the curtain cord to reveal a brass plaque to commemorate the occasion. It was a poignant moment when Deborah cut the ribbon. After fourteen years Frances's dream of a national purpose built training centre had finally come true.

The Frances Hay Centre was given a Royal seal of approval on April 1, 2003 when Princess Anne accepted Peter Gorbing's invitation to visit the centre and unveil a plaque to commemorate the charity's fifteenth anniversary. Lady Juliet Townsend, the Lord Lieutenant of Northamptonshire and the Queen's representative in the county, introduced the Princess Royal to the trustees, president and chief executive. After signing the visitors' book members of the Royal party enjoyed an introduction to the charity's work, a tour of the accommodation block and a series of demonstrations, the first of which was a puppy class.

The Princess also met several clients and their dogs. Byron and Gill Harvey explained how their dog Isis worked for both of them, Dick Thomsett told her how his life had changed since Pippa came into it and young Jamie Sutherland showed how he grooms and cares for his dog Kandy.

Princess Anne was also interested in finding out about the fundraising process and chatted with volunteer fundraiser Maureen Goulden, who offered the Royal visitor a chance to win a cuddly mascot.

Maureen said afterwards: 'At first the Princess was worried that her dogs would destroy any toys but eventually she chose a HERO mascot and wished us all the best in our fundraising.'

A Royal visit – another first for the charity and something else that Frances Hay would have been proud of.

Chapter five
Twice the blessings

Byron and Gill Harvey were teenage sweethearts. They met when they were sixteen and married three years later. By their early fifties they were just the same as any other long-married couple approaching middle age. With full lives and varied interests, they spent their free time in the garden and enjoyed the company of their dog, a flirty young lady named Isis.

Just the same as other couples? Well no, not exactly. Byron and Gill both relied totally on wheelchairs for their mobility, whether in their Nottinghamshire home or when they were out and about. Byron's disability is the result of polio when he was a toddler, which left him with spondylosis in his neck and back as well as a damaged spine. Gill was born with spina bifida, but refused to let it get in the way of living an active life. She was a great walker and enjoyed doing things for herself and for Byron. For a while, Byron feels, he was the bigger problem. He suffered a great deal of pain, which wore him down. Sadly, because of ill health, Gill had to retire from work in 1992. A year later Byron, too, had to give up his job and his mood darkened. Then in 1994, when Gill was 42, tragedy struck. She had to have both legs amputated above the knee because of poor circulation and was permanently confined to a wheelchair as a result.

Despite this, Byron says that disability for him was 'just normal life', although it was clearly harder for Gill after her operation. They were both grateful to have had parents who made them get on with things as children and teenagers.

'Two weeks before I left school my Dad said "Don't ever let anyone tell you you can't do it," said Byron. 'That's how I got my first job as an electronics engineer at Plessey.

'They were dubious about taking me on but that was red rag to a bull as far as I was concerned. I asked them to give me just the same opportunity as anyone else. I didn't want any favours and I didn't want any special treatment, just three months to prove myself. I finally left after 24 years! I think the key to combating disability is in your head. You have to make the most of what you've got. My motto is you only get one shot at life.'

After Gill lost her legs the couple did their best to carry on as usual but life was not easy.

'When two of you are disabled it's a different ball game. Even simple things like changing a light bulb or getting things from high cupboards become impossible, because neither of you can do them,' said Byron.

So it was a great day in their lives when, in August 1995, they were given the chance to be the first couple to share an assistance dog from Dogs for the Disabled.

They had never even heard of the charity until a few months previously. A keen caravaner, Byron was at the Caravan and Boat Show at the NEC in Birmingham.

'Guide dogs had a stand there with a few retired dogs and after I'd fussed over the dogs I got talking to the man on the stand. He told me about Dogs for the Disabled, got me the information and we applied.'

Their unique partnership began with Bianca, a German shepherd bitch who proved to be a willing helper and a great companion. Not only that, with Bianca's arrival Byron noticed his pain diminished and his stress levels dropped.

'When you're in a wheelchair you do drop things and it's a killer having to pick them up. It's not that you can't do it; it's the pain when you do. The dog made such a difference.'

Sadly though, the couple's pleasure in their new friend was short-lived. A few months later Bianca had an ear infection, followed by surgery, which permanently damaged her hearing. Dogs for the Disabled took the difficult decision to retire Bianca and she went to live with Carole Cluett in Poole, Dorset.

Then Anton arrived. Gill and Byron were delighted to have another dog and Anton was worth his weight in gold to them. In October 1997 a film crew from BBC television's *Rolf's Amazing World of Animals* descended on Kirkby in Ashfield to film Byron, Gill and Anton and the following February they were invited to the studio to film with Rolf Harris – they even had their own dressing room, with their names above the door. The programme was screened the following summer, when Rolf told the audience, 'These dogs are extraordinary. There is nothing more joyful than watching them, both at work and at play'.

But two years later Byron and Gill were again faced with

the pain of parting with their best friend. Anton was
diagnosed with cancer and although an operation to remove
a lump was successful he began to find work stressful and
the charity decided to retire him in January 2001. Anton has
gone on to enjoy a good long life with Fiona Briglmen and is
still with her today.

A few weeks later Byron and Gill were back at the
training centre with Tom, the young, glossy black Labrador
who had won hearts during the official opening ceremony of
the Frances Hay Centre by pulling the cord to unveil a
commemorative plaque. He was so pleased with the applause
this generated that he pulled the cord again, and again, and
again ...

Beautiful and clever as Tom was, however, his
partnership with Gill and Byron was short-lived. Their
garden was a low-maintenance paved area and Tom was
used to grass. He refused to relieve himself on hard ground,
a distressing problem for all concerned. He went back to the
training centre to see if the difficulty could be put right, but
to no avail. Tom went off to retrain – successfully – with
another client who has a grassy garden but Byron and Gill
were again dogless and there were some long and painful
months before another suitable dog came along for them.

'Tom was a beautiful dog and between us we tried
everything. But he needed grass and we got rid of ours ten
years earlier as it was impossible for us to look after it. In
the months after Tom went we realised that having an
assistance dog is not only helpful but also very rewarding
and it helped us to appreciate how much pressure and pain

the dog takes away from everyday life,' said Byron.

Eventually, though, the right dog came along and they were matched with Isis, a blue blooded Golden Retriever who took her name from the goddess of Egyptian mythology. She settled well with her new partners and proved to be an exceptional assistance dog, working equally as well for Byron as for Gill. Isis was trained to do all the usual things, such as helping with dressing and undressing, opening and closing doors, emptying the washing machine and making light of pegging out the washing. But she also did two things that were unique to her. One was to swap the couple's newspaper from one to the other when they ask her to and the other was to fetch Gill's wheelchair for her: Byron and Gill had a large television and when they settled down to watch their favourite programmes Gill had to push her wheelchair out of the way so that Byron could see the screen properly. When Gill needed her chair again, Isis fetched it by pulling on a lead that was attached to it, and positioning it within Gill's reach.

Isis was the first dog to have been trained by Dogs for the Disabled specifically to work with two people but she coped well and showed no sign of divided loyalties. Lots of dogs have individual preferences for men or women and there was no doubt that Isis was a 'ladies' dog'. If she wanted fuss and cuddles she instinctively turned to Gill but when it came to work she shared her favours equally between her owners.

But whatever the instructors say about not letting a dog rule the roost, Byron says Isis was the leader of their little pack.

'When you've got a working dog you have to put her first and think of her before yourself. For instance, we were going on a Mediterranean cruise and could have had Isis vaccinated and taken her with us. It would certainly have made our lives easier if we did. But we believed it would not have been in her best interest to go so we managed without her on our holiday and she had a holiday with Jean & Fred Nicholls, her puppy socialisers. Now aged nine, she still goes to Jean and Fred for her holidays.

Byron and Gill had 32 years of happy marriage and the shared pleasure of their beloved assistance dogs until 2004, when Gill died suddenly of a massive heart attack.

Grief stricken, Byron turned to Sue McCarthy, an old friend of both Gill and Byron, whose assistance dog Inka was the twin to Isis.

Sue, who was divorced, has had many life threatening illnesses. She has been severely disabled and in a wheelchair since 1994, when she contracted spinal bacterial meningitis, a condition that left her unable to do the simplest of everyday tasks for herself.

She struggled to maintain her independence but things came to a head after she went shopping, got caught in the rain and was trapped in her wet raincoat for three hours before plucking up the courage to ask for some help from a passer by. This left her exhausted and depressed. She went to bed too tired to get undressed and slept fully clothed. She really didn't want to wake up and struggle on but her son Ross went to see her and told her about Dogs for the Disabled. Later the same day she made contact with the charity and a few months later she was partnered with Inka, at about the same time that Byron and Gill were matched with Isis.

The three humans struck up a strong friendship and the two golden retrievers maintained their sisterly bonds. All of a sudden there was light for Sue at the end of a long dark tunnel.

'I was desperate to get somebody to help me dress and undress and suddenly, here was this amazing dog who did exactly this, and much more, even down to picking things up as small as tiny earrings. We were a team.

'Inka totally transformed my life and I am now a different person. Human beings get tired of being carers but dogs never do. No matter how many times you drop something they are always happy to pick it up. It is a great game to them.'

But twelve months after Gill's death Inka developed a fast growing cancer and on January 29, 2007 she had to be put to sleep. Sue was devastated. She turned to Byron for comfort and he was only too pleased to help, especially as Sue had given him months of endless support day and night.

After several months Sue was partnered with Max, another golden retriever, although she was still heartbroken about her beloved Inka. She and Byron continued to support each other through the dark days and gradually, as their grief lessened, their friendship turned to romance and then love.

On 7th June 2008, St Mary's Church in a small market town in Oxfordshire was packed with family, friends and well wishers for Sue and Byron's wedding. The couple and their dogs have made their home in Thame, the town where they married.

Isis and Max are special to Dogs for the Disabled because they have shown how kind, reward-based training can teach dogs to work with a couple just as well as with one person. But the two dogs are special to Byron and Sue in other ways too.

'They allow us to keep our independence. When you're in a wheelchair for some 40 or 50 years, you don't get blasé. The older you get, the harder everyday tasks get, for example when doing the washing, gardening and shopping

'So having an assistance dog helps to decrease pain levels and provides something else to think about, rather than your own pain and problems. Isis and Max are so finely tuned in to us that they know if we are having a bad day – we don't have to tell them, they just know. They know instinctively what we want, such as when we drop things and they pick them up without us having to ask them to.

'Another thing is that people are more sociable and friendly towards us because of the dogs. Shopping trips take twice as long these days as people want to chat about our wonderful dogs. Isis and Max are really laid back and take us in their stride. They are both absolute stars and they really are our best friends. Dogs for the Disabled really do change lives. They certainly have helped change ours in more ways than one.'

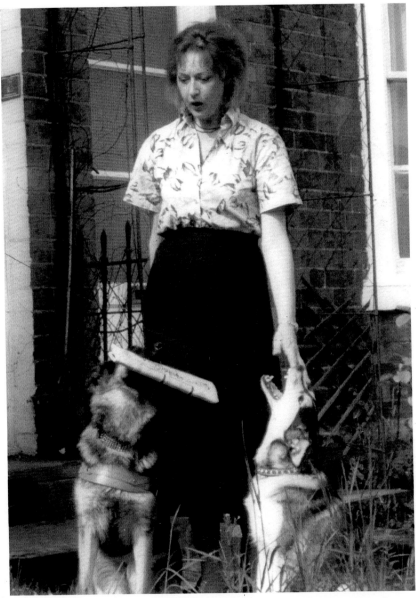

A rare photograph of Frances Hay, Dogs for the Disabled's founder. Pic: Dogs for the Disabled

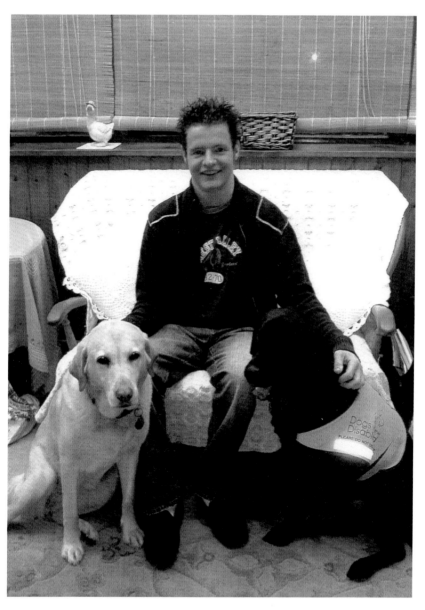

Jamie Sutherland with his retired dog, Kandy (left) and her successor, Tyler. Pic: Jamie Sutherland

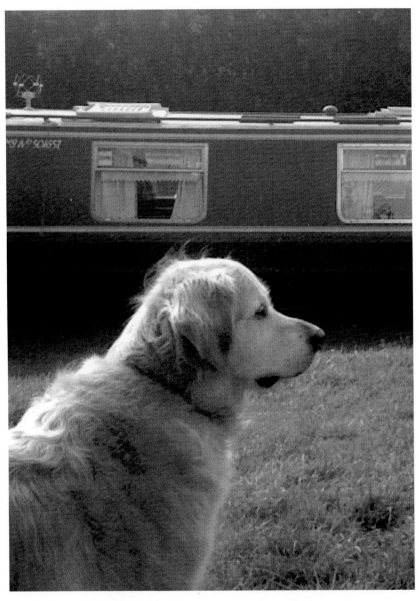

Caesar – even after nine years as an assistance dog he's still keen to try out new experiences. Pic: Wendy Morrell

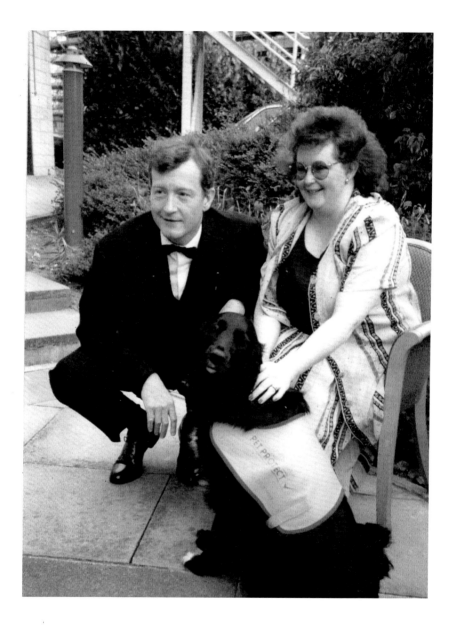

Sarah with Jade and snooker ace Steve Davis.
Pic: Martin Carr

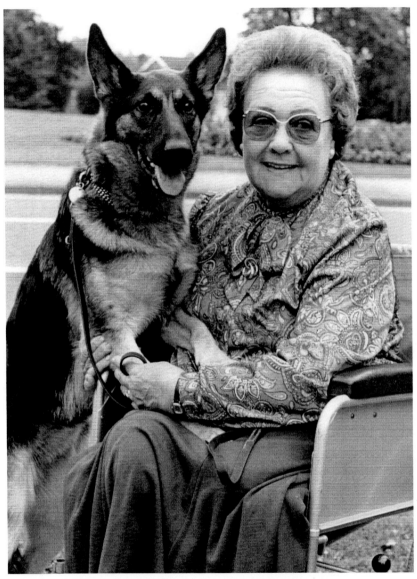

Gladys Rainbow with Rani – the UK's first assistance dog.
Pic: Coventry Evening Telegraph, by kind permission of
Geoff Rainbow

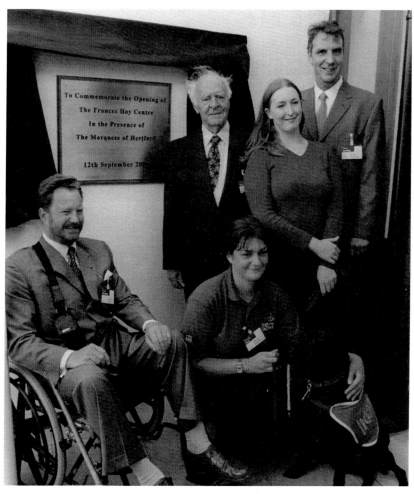

The formal opening of The Frances Hay Centre.
Clockwise from left: Lord Hertford, the charity's patron;
George Newns and Deborah Hay, Frances Hay's father and
daughter; Peter Gorbing, Dogs for the Disabled's chief
executive; instructor Louise Hart with Tom.
Pic: Marc Henrie, by kind permission of Dogs for the
Disabled

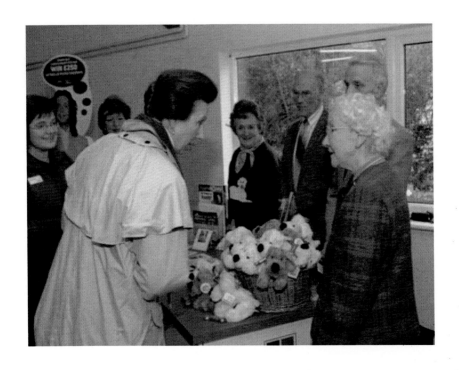

The Princess Royal meets volunteer Maureen Goulden and a collection of HERO mascots. Pic: Dogs for the Disabled

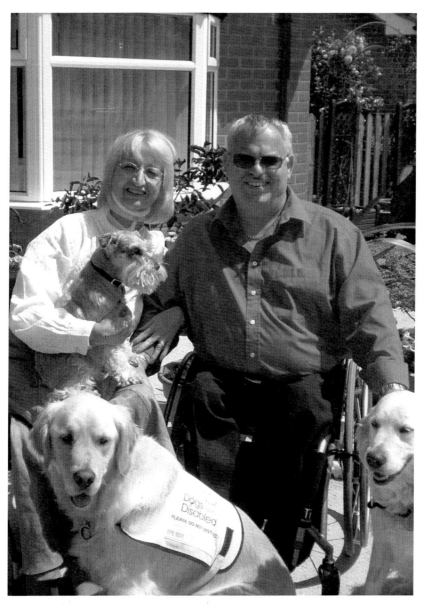

Byron and Sue Harvey with pet dog Daisy and assistance dogs Max and Isis. Pic: Sue and Byron Harvey

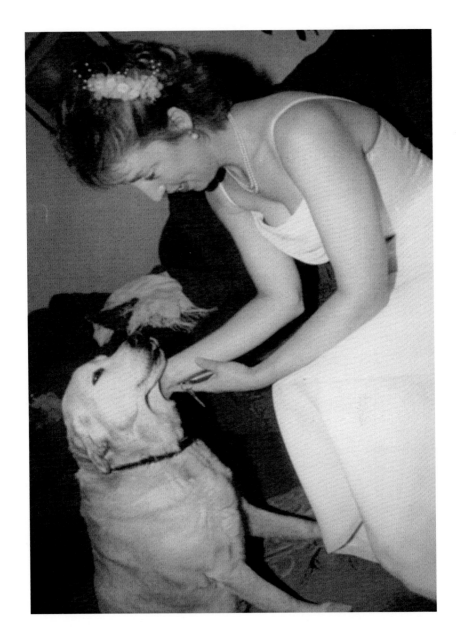

Zane with Corrine on her wedding day. Pic: Corrine Mitchell

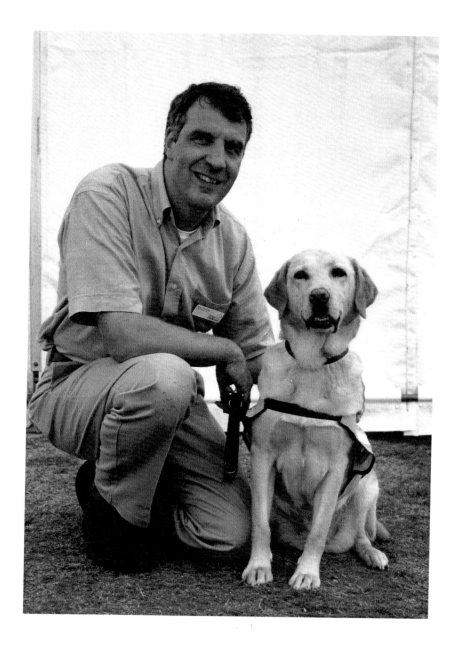

Chief Executive Peter Gorbing. Pic: Dogs for the Disabled

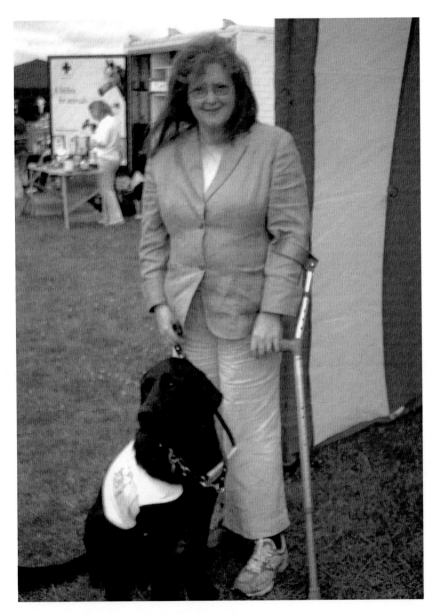

Sarah with Demi, her new best friend.
Pic: Sarah's private collection

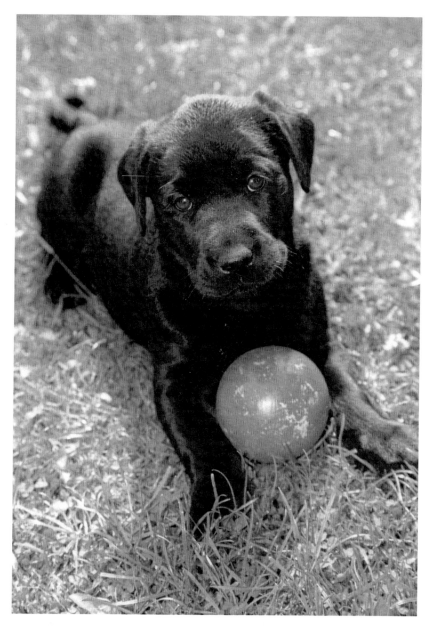

Puppy playtime. Pic: Dogs for the Disabled

Chapter six
Training is fun

Training a dog to qualify as an assistant for a disabled
person is a long and intensive process. Ideally, puppies with
an eye on a career as assistance dogs should start being
socialised from the age of six weeks. This means getting
them used to as many situations as possible, ready for when
they have to face them in their working lives. As the puppies
grow older they are introduced to such things as meeting
people and other animals, public transport, shopping centres,
lorries with noisy air brakes, travelling in cars and being left
on their own for short periods, all of which will help them to
be relaxed and comfortable with almost any situation they
may meet during their working lives. In addition, they learn
basic obedience and the beginnings of good social behaviour,
including toileting on command. On top of all this, they also
get used to being groomed and having routine health checks
of their eyes, ears and teeth, as well as that bone of
contention for many pet dogs, visiting the vet!

These skills all lay the vital groundwork that is necessary
for the later, highly complex training and development of a
happy, well adjusted and obedient assistance dog. It was
with this in mind that Dogs for the Disabled realised the
importance of starting the dogs' training while they were

still young and the charity launched its successful puppy socialising scheme in September 1997. Within four years there were 30 volunteer puppy socialisers within a one-hour drive of the charity's national headquarters near Banbury, and the scheme continues to grow.

Because the puppies' informal training starts at such a young age they are out and about much earlier than most dogs and therefore their vaccination programme also begins earlier than usual.

Before any of this can happen, however, the most important step of all has to be taken, and that is the selection of the puppy. Although rescued dogs were used in the early days of the charity, the failure rate was quite high. This was because too little was known about the dogs' background and breeding and it soon became clear that there was a higher chance of success with dogs that had been specially bred for the purpose. Working dogs with a long family history of being trained for a specific purpose are more likely to produce puppies who are equally up to the task and so these days Dogs for the Disabled looks at dogs' pedigrees as part of the selection process. Because training is so intensive it costs a great deal of money to teach a dog to work in partnership with a disabled person and, admirable though it was to give abandoned dogs a purpose in life, the charity had to recognise that rescue dogs would not form a reliable source.

The Guide Dogs for the Blind Association, or GDBA, proved to be a real support. They began to provide Dogs for the Disabled with dogs that, once they had started training, were found to be unsuitable as guide dogs. One common reason for this was that a dog was not 'forward going' enough. A guide dog has to lead, or walk in front of its handler, but not all dogs are happy doing this. Assistance dogs, on the other hand, are often expected to walk sedately alongside a wheelchair and many of the dogs donated by GDBA had this type of personality. Until a few years ago, a third of Dogs for the Disabled's qualified dogs started their training as guide dogs and the majority went on to become successful assistance dogs.

More recently, however, Dogs for the Disabled started its own breeding programme and at the same time its instructors began to select puppies from a variety of carefully chosen breeders whose animals have good track records as working dogs. The most commonly used breeds are purebred golden retrievers and Labrador retrievers because of their natural ability to retrieve and their willingness to learn. A first cross from these two breeds also produces some very good dogs. Other breeds can also be ideal. For example, the charity has successfully trained a Leonberger, a large strong and muscular breed with a confident calmness that makes them ideal for clients who need help with balance and stability. It has also been successful with a Finnish Lapphund, a much smaller breed that is ideal for people who may be physically frail. Lapphunds were only imported into the UK in 1989 but this strongly built, brave and faithful little dog has been used by the Lapps in Finland for hundreds of years to herd reindeer. Intelligent, willing, calm and affectionate, they make ideal assistance dogs.

Members of the dog supply team know from feedback exactly what qualities to look for in puppies but their first step is to study the pedigrees from previous successful matings and check whether there will be a repeat mating between the dog and bitch concerned. Once they have identified a possible litter a dog selector visits the puppies when they are 'in the nest' and again when they are about six to seven weeks old. During this visit they put the pups into a number of different situations, such as noise, and assess their reactions. They want to see, for example, how responsive the puppies are and whether they will retrieve a small article.

'Even at this age you can learn a lot about a puppy's personality,' said the dog selectors.

They handle and play with the puppies individually so that by the end of the visit they have a good idea about which of the puppies are likely to take to training. This is also the time when the dog selectors are able to judge whether the puppies are trusting or nervous, gentle or aggressive.

When a selected puppy is seven weeks old and the dog selectors are satisfied that it meets all the criteria, it is placed in the care of a carefully chosen volunteer puppy socialiser where it lives as a member of the family for the next twelve to fourteen months. If the socialiser is new to the job the puppy coordinator may make two or three visits in quick succession so that any early problems can be sorted out. Otherwise the puppy coordinator will carry out regular assessments and is always on hand to offer help, advice and support to the puppy's foster family.

Regular puppy classes are held at The Frances Hay Centre or near to the socialisers' homes if they are based in a satellite area. This gives socialisers and puppies a chance to mix with each other, share their experiences and generally have an enjoyable time together, as well as learning new skills at the same time.

The role of puppy socialiser is a vital one and one which lays the foundation for the dog's future. Jean Nicholls is experienced at socialising Dogs for the Disabled puppies and loves to talk about what the job involves. Her role is to provide a secure, loving environment for the puppy but there is more to it than that. While the young dogs are in the socialisers' care they are expected to learn basic obedience, to be clean indoors and to respond to the dog whistle, both outside and as a signal to begin eating at mealtimes.

'But,' says Jean, 'most importantly, the dogs must learn to be good mixers and be comfortable in all kinds of situations. To do this I gradually introduce them to as many different environments as possible, such as going to a school, a church or a park. I teach them to walk to heel on a lead, to mix with other dogs and to be happy when children are around.'

By the time a puppy is seven months old it will be making regular visits to busy towns and shopping centres, going in and out of lifts, visiting train and bus stations, pubs and restaurants. Throughout this time, right up to the moment the puppy qualifies as an assistance dog, it wears a distinctive green jacket so that everyone can see this is no ordinary puppy.

Puppy socialising is something the whole family can be involved with. Jean says she and her family have a lot of fun with their 'foster puppies', although she worried about how she would cope when it was time for their first puppy to leave home and join the grown up world of trainee assistance dogs.

'Of course', she says, 'when the day came it was tinged with sadness because we were parting with a much-loved friend. But we all felt very proud as well, because we knew we had played an important part in helping to improve the quality of life for a disabled person.'

Training begins in earnest at around twelve months of age, when the young dog leaves the puppy socialiser and returns to the training centre. Once there it is assigned to one of the charity's trainers for a six-week assessment, during which time it is monitored in a variety of situations. This enables the trainer to build up a picture of the dog's strengths and weaknesses. The dog is never put under any pressure – everything is a big game and the training sessions are short, so the young recruit is always eager to please and willing to learn, with no loss of enthusiasm.

All the puppy socialisers receive a report on 'their' puppy's progress after its first assessment and many of them continue to keep in touch throughout the dog's working life.

Dogs for the Disabled is a leader in the field of training assistance dogs. All the dogs are trained with an emphasis on play and by making the most of their natural pulling and retrieving instincts. They are always rewarded for good behaviour, either with praise, food, fuss or a free run. Unwanted behaviour is never punished, simply ignored.

After the dog has been assessed and the trainer is satisfied that it has what it takes to become an assistance dog, the next stage of training begins. This lasts around three months. With encouragement from the trainer the dog becomes confident in basic obedience, social behaviour, heelwork and carrying out tasks on command.

Once a dog has mastered all these skills it moves on to a more advanced level of training, in readiness for working with a disabled partner. At this level the instructor encourages the dog to take greater responsibility for its actions, ready for the final stage of training when it is matched with a disabled person and meets its future partner for the first time. Matching is a very important process and one that is handled with great care and sensitivity by the instructors. After all, the dog and its human will be enjoying a very close and special relationship for many years so it is vitally important that they get on well together and respond positively to each other. Once the partnership has been matched the dog is trained to meet the specific needs of the client, whether it is to pick up things that have been dropped, to bark for attention in an emergency, to aid balance or to help with the shopping or laundry. This highly specialised training usually lasts four to six weeks and, as always, is reward focused so that the dog always enjoys itself.

Eventually the time comes for human and canine to renew their earlier brief acquaintance and begin the unique partnership-training course that will set them on the road to a happy, mutually fulfilling and interdependent life together.

This two-week course is designed in such a way that the instructor gives one hundred per cent support to client and dog. The objectives are to send the client home with a good knowledge of dog welfare, dog psychology and the commands to be used. It is also important for the client to go home feeling safe and confident, even though most of them are a little nervous to begin with. It is a big step to leave the security of the training centre after two weeks, to be alone with your new charge and solely responsible for its well-being.

The client doesn't have any contact with the dog until the second day of the course, to give the human participant a chance to settle in and to revise the ten most-used commands. During the course clients also learn how to motivate their four-legged partner as well as themselves.

There is also time for some role-play involving the instructor and the client, when the instructor becomes the dog. This enables the client to put commands into practice, by trying them out for the first few times on a 'human canine'. This naturally looks very amusing and raises a few laughs to start with but it has a serious, and positive, side too because it enables clients to gain confidence in giving commands before they have to try it out on the dog.

Finally the big moment arrives, when the dog is handed over to the client. Imagine you are that client. You sit nervously in your room waiting for the knock on the door and wondering if the dog will like you, listen to you or even respond to you. After what seems like an eternity the instructor enters with your new best friend. The hand-over is done as calmly and quietly as possible and then you are alone with your dog. It is time to get to know each other. From this moment on you are responsible for the feeding and welfare of your dog. Life will never be the same again!

A new partnership receives training in several different environments during the next couple of weeks. Sometimes the pair will go to a shopping precinct or a supermarket. It can be a daunting experience for both partners to go into a busy place for the first time, and the instructor carefully monitors the reactions of both of them in any new situation.

At the end of the fortnight the dog and client return home to begin a new life together. Known as home placement, this is the time for the two of them to put into practice everything they learnt during their training and to start with they receive intensive support from their instructor. The dog is introduced slowly to its new surroundings inside and outside the home. This usually includes visiting shops used by the client and, more importantly from a dog's point of view, the local park – they always seem to have the uncanny knack of sniffing out just where their nearest free running area is and the quickest way of getting to it!

The pair also visits the local veterinary surgery for the first six-monthly check up, an occasion that the vets always do their best to make as pleasant as possible by offering the dog a small treat. This encourages the dog to think the vet's is a very nice place to visit.

At this point in training the support from the instructor is reduced to allow the client to take over as the dog's trainer. Although the instructors make fewer visits they continue to monitor the new partnership closely. Once they are satisfied that everything is working well they arrange for the training manager, or director of training to visit and observe the partnership in action. If the client is confident and competent with the dog, inside and outside the home, the partnership is then qualified. The client signs a contract and hands over a nominal fee to adopt the dog, who is rewarded with a bright yellow qualifying jacket and lots of well-deserved praise.

Dogs for the Disabled can help people with a wide range of physical disabilities such as those brought about by multiple sclerosis, cerebral palsy, strokes, arthritis, polio, spina bifida and accidents to maintain a good level of independence. Anyone over the age of sixteen who can demonstrate a need for an assistance dog, is resident in England or Wales and is self-motivated can apply. The only criteria is that the dog should be able to do for you some of the things you are unable to do for yourself, and you must be able to look after the dog properly by yourself.

The yellow jacket worn by qualified assistance dogs carries Dogs for the Disabled's logo as well as the logo of Assistance Dogs UK. This is an umbrella organisation that promotes high standards of training, behaviour and hygiene for all assistance dogs in the United Kingdom. These include guide dogs, hearing dogs, dogs for disabled people and support dogs for people who have conditions such as epilepsy. All clients carry an accredited Ministry of Health card, which means the dogs meet the required high standard of health and hygiene needed to enter restaurants and food shops.

If all goes well, the working life of a Dog for the Disabled dog is approximately eight to ten years. When the dog reaches its tenth birthday the workload is reduced and the instructors begin to think about finding the client a successor dog. Ideally, the retired dog remains with the client and becomes a role model for the young recruit. This is not always possible, however, and on these occasions the instructor turns to the charity's waiting list of people who are eager to give a retired dog a well-earned rest and several happy golden years of retirement.

Chapter seven

Retirement – Zane's story

They say life begins at retirement but I wasn't really sure what to expect. You know what it's like. You've been busy all your life and suddenly, retirement looms.

What was I going to do? I couldn't sit in the house all day. I'd get fat and lazy, and anyway there's nothing on the telly. Take up a new hobby? Travel the world? Well I did none of these but I did get a new owner... and that changed my world completely.

I had been a working dog with Dogs for the Disabled for some years when "they" decided it was time I had a rest. First, though, they had to find me a suitable home, no easy decision. I needed space for my belongings, my own room to relax in and I didn't want to be bothered by noisy youngsters.

Eventually I found the ideal place near Bicester, in Oxfordshire, where there are fields nearby for when I feel like going for a walk. The accommodation is reasonable, too. There's a large garden with a well stocked fish pond, plenty of thick rugs to lie on and lots of visitors who can always be persuaded to give me a nice juicy treat whenever Corrine, my new human, isn't looking. She was a police officer but when I came along she decided to work part-time, which is much better for us both.

Of course, being a lazy Labrador, I'd planned on a nice quiet retirement. You know the sort of thing: gentle ambles around the park, lots of fuss while I laze in front of the fire, choc drops for pudding – but I was in for a shock!

It started with a scuba-diving trip to Leicestershire, to a flooded quarry. Corrine and her friends dressed up in some strange smelling outfits, put on lots of weird looking contraptions, jumped into the water and disappeared from view. I had to keep watch and chase the ducks away from the water's edge until they came out again. The best bit was that while Corrine was in the water I was able to persuade lots of people to share their bacon rolls with me – it's amazing what humans will do when you gaze into their eyes and wag your tail at them.

The next surprise was when we visited the Brecon Beacons, which was where I discovered sheep. I don't know why but Corrine decided to put me on the lead while we were there. Spoilsport! Then we climbed a mountain and I have a lovely photograph of Corrine and me at the top.

As well as all this I've been to college with Corrine on her horticultural course – more bacon rolls – and I always check out the gardens she works on, for the softest grass and neighbouring cats.

So as you can see, my life is very full. Retirement is certainly different from what I expected but I've made some great new friends and done lots of new things. So when your turn comes, don't worry about it. Just go out there and have fun!

Corrine takes up the story.

In 2001 Zane developed a problem with his left shoulder. He had an x-ray and the condition was diagnosed as arthritis. The area was swollen and obviously painful for him, although it had no effect on his rear end – the tail still wagged enthusiastically at the least little thing!

The vet prescribed some medicine for him and the effects were quite dramatic. He was bouncing around like a puppy again and the swelling went down. He stayed on the tablets for a couple of months then came off them but had to go back on them a few months later, on a higher dose, when the swelling and pain recurred. Unfortunately, insuring a dog after the age of ten is very expensive so Zane was no longer insured but luckily Dogs for the Disabled helped with the costs. At £40 a month for the tablets alone, it was getting to be a struggle.

This time the swelling never really went away. Zane struggled to get out of the car and jumping down was obviously getting harder. It made his shoulder worse and because of this he was having to stay at home more often. However he was still the happy dog that everyone loved. It was clear that he was getting older and needed to slow down.

By summer 2002 the swelling was getting worse and Zane went back for a check-up. This time the vet thought he might have a tumour on his shoulder.

'What can be done for that?' I asked. After a pause, the vet replied, 'Amputate the limb'. I was horrified. At Zane's age, there was no way he would be able to cope. So the decision was made to let nature take its course. Zane was quite old by now and had had a loving and enjoyable life. I was not going to put him through any additional pain. His dosage was increased and he seemed content.

In November I married and we planned our honeymoon for December: four weeks in Australia, visiting friends and touring around. What were we to do with Zane? My husband's parents agreed to come and stay with Zane for the first two weeks then he would go to stay with a friend nearby, where he had stayed before. However, I was worried. He was slowing down considerably on his walks, which were now just a short stroll around the park next to our house. And he was struggling to get in and out of the car, even though I now put him on the rear seats rather than in the boot.

A week before we were due to fly out, the decision was made for us. Zane enthusiastically headed out of the door for his walk but only got twenty yards before stopping. I was in tears as I walked him slowly back home. We had always said that when he could not go for his walk it was time to call it a day. I called the vet and tearfully requested an appointment for the next day.

That night we spent hugging Zane who thought it was wonderful, all this attention! We talked through the options but knew that there was no real alternative. There had been no treatment for his tumour and it was time to let him go before it got too painful for him. It is the most difficult decision to make – when do you let go of your faithful companion? We did not want to delay the inevitable for our own sakes, so that we did not have to make that decision. Even now, I worried whether we were doing it for the wrong reasons, because we were going away. However I could not give the decision to someone else – that would not have been fair. And we knew that although Zane would have been well looked after, he would have been very upset at being left.

The next day, we took Zane to the vet's. My husband was so upset that he could not come in and so I took Zane in for his last appointment. The vet confirmed that there really was little we could do to help him any more and so I sat on the floor holding him while the injection was readied. Zane was quite calm, just looking at me, wondering what all the fuss was about.

It was so quick. Zane continued to gaze into my eyes as the injection was given. His eyes closed and he was gone.

Zane gave me nearly four years of immense pleasure. He was so happy with life and everyone who met him loved him. I am very grateful that we were able to spend those years together. I shall never forget him.

Corrine Mitchell

Chapter eight
Who pays?

Raising funds is vital to Dogs for the Disabled's survival. The charity receives no Government funding and has to generate income so that it can continue to train dogs as Frances Hay would have wished. Put simply: no money, no dogs.

Fundraising is fun and there are many ways of going about it. The dynamic fundraising team employed at the charity's headquarters is supported by a dedicated band of volunteers who work tirelessly to spread the word of Dogs for the Disabled.

For example, individual registered speakers give talks about the charity to schools, clubs and a wide range of professional and commercial organisations. These people believe passionately in their subject, especially as many of them are clients with dogs. They all have their own stories to tell and view their efforts as a way of giving something back to the charity and a way of saying thank you for their newfound confidence and independence.

There is also a network of community fundraising groups around the country. Group members spend many of their weekends at fetes, street collections and boot sales, as well as arranging their own money-spinning activities.

One of the largest events to be staged by a volunteer group was held in Warwickshire in 2000. The supporters' group in the county decided to hold a sponsored walk in Abbey Fields, Kenilworth to celebrate the millennium and to commemorate the tenth anniversary of Frances Hay's death by dedicating a bench in her memory.

The date was set for May 21 and although the organisers knew what an enormous task they had taken on they were determined it would be a success. Thanks to people's generosity they received enough donations to pay for a bench and plaque in Abbey Fields, even before the walk got underway.

On the morning of the walk everyone awoke to the sound of rain beating against the window. Hearts sank. Eighteen months of planning could be ruined by the weather. But the despondency was short lived. Despite the rain people started arriving and setting up their stalls. It was exciting to see the 'Walk on the Wild Side' come together for real.

The sun began to shine and the local Cubbington Silver Band began to play. The then Mayor of Kenilworth, Councillor Graham Windybank, and other invited guests then gathered for the unveiling of the Frances Hay bench. This was carried out by Fran's father, George Newns, while her daughter Deborah looked on. Mr Newns said that no-one who knew Frances would ever forget her.

'She was a wonderful person with a sense of humour and an infectious laugh – I can hear it now.

'Founding Dogs for the Disabled was no easy task. Frances had no capital, only herself, her dog and an idea.

Her problems were brushed aside by her qualities of determination and enthusiasm.

'She had a dream that one day there would be training centres throughout the country to serve disabled people. That dream is beginning to come true and it is very sad she is not here today to see it.

'Frances had only one wish, that when the charity was big and successful that she would be remembered as starting it all. I am proud to be her father and to be unveiling this bench in memory of her pioneering work.'

It was poignant to hear that Frances always wanted to be remembered for starting the charity and fitting to have a lasting memorial in Abbey Fields, which was one of her favourite places. Members of the Warwickshire Supporters' Group felt honoured to have played a part in fulfilling her wishes.

Peter Purves, the former Blue Peter presenter and until recently the BBC's senior commentator at Crufts dog show, travelled from his home in Suffolk especially to start the sponsored walk. He gave a warm speech before cutting the ribbon and sending dogs and walkers on their way. One hundred people of all ages took part in the walk around the ornamental lake in Abbey Fields, the sun continued to shine and the event raised more than £3,500 for Dogs for the Disabled.

Another event to raise a large sum of money was attended by Dogs for the Disabled client Kate Tudor-Hart from Plymouth and her dog Kris. Every August the Kenn Charter Fayre is held in Devon. The Fayre, which dates from 900AD, goes back to the days of King Offa of Mercia, who used it as a means of collecting tithes from the villagers of Kenn, Kennford and Chapham. The principal of raising money has not been forgotten and these days it is used to raise cash for worthwhile causes. Around £5,000 was raised in August 2001 and the money was shared between Dogs for the Disabled, Exeter Hospiscare and other local charities.

Natalie Cornah, a presenter with BBC TV in Plymouth, opened the Fayre. Later the two celebrities, Natalie and Kris, were happy to pose for photographs together. Kris, like all the charity's dogs, is used to making the most of every opportunity to raise people's awareness of Dogs for the Disabled.

In the days leading up to the Fayre, villagers were treated to the modern pantomime Rumpelstiltskin.com, a murder mystery evening and an auction, which raised £1,000. Anthea Turner donated an autographed keep-fit video, and Wendy Richard donated an Albert Square sign, autographed by the cast of EastEnders.

Dogs for the Disabled has enjoyed good media coverage over the years. Its first appearance on Blue Peter was in 1989 when client Amanda Knapp visited the studio with Poppy, who was happy to show off her skills on Amanda's command and was quite unfazed by the studio set up. Amanda and Poppy later featured in the 25th Anniversary edition of the Blue Peter Annual.

Blue Peter also filmed another client, Ann Greenwood, and her dog Shep on location around their home near

Bodmin. Ann keeps horses and Shep was keen to show the Blue Peter team just what he could do. As well as opening and closing farm gates his special job was to go under a horse's belly, pick up the girth strap and give it to Ann to fasten. This is quite a challenge for any dog but for Shep, an appealing Border collie, it was a real triumph. As a young dog he'd been thrown out of a van on the M6 and was rescued by friends of Frances Hay who saw what had happened. Shep was living proof that despite a shaky start in life a dog can overcome its fears to lead a happy and fulfilling life, given praise, affection and encouragement.

The film crew returned in January 1998 to catch up with Ann and Shep and new recruit Baron. Shep was retiring because of his sensitivity to noise, so Ann needed a replacement dog. Shep continued to live with Ann until his death in October 2002 and was a good role model for Baron, a large German Shepherd, who was quick and willing to learn the tasks that were required of him every day.

Baron was half way through his training when Blue Peter presenter Connie Huq visited. Ann uses the same clicker training technique as the Dogs for the Disabled trainers and instructors use for all the dogs. Every time Baron did something right Ann clicked and gave him a treat. She ignored any unwanted behaviour so that Baron associated the click with a reward and was willing to repeat the exercise again and again. He was happy to demonstrate some of his new skills to Connie. Ann asked Baron to pull off her sock and as soon as he did she clicked and gave him a treat. Baron also showed how he could collect the newspaper from the letterbox, remove washing from the machine and pick up the phone.

Ann's favourite way of getting to the village is by pony and trap. During the programme Dogs for the Disabled instructor Carolyn Bull met Ann, Baron and Connie outside the post office where Baron got a chance to learn another new skill. Carolyn took Baron to meet the postmaster, who called Baron up to the counter and gave him a few treats. After they had made friends, Carolyn gave Baron Ann's wallet to pass over the counter and after another reward Baron happily returned the wallet to Ann who was waiting outside.

Dogs for the Disabled was chosen to appear on BBC's Lifeline appeal programme in 1996, when Wendy Richard made the appeal on behalf of the charity. She went to visit Janet Turner and Verney and saw how Janet used a special harness on Verney, to steady her when walking. Janet has cerebral palsy and Verney gave her the confidence to go out on her own and feel safe. The appeal also featured other clients and their dogs and was a huge success, raising £63,000 from viewers.

Four years later the BBC selected Dogs for the Disabled for a second Lifeline appeal. Annette Crosbie launched the appeal this time and met Jill Brown and her dog Astrid. Jill explained how she was able to live independently in her own home because she knew Astrid would fetch the things she needed, from shoes and splints to the post. Astrid even helped Jill undress by pulling her jacket and socks off.

Before Jill had a dog she rarely went out. Her deteriorating bone condition means she has to wear splints and a neck brace, and people were too embarrassed to look at her or speak to her. Because she uses a wheelchair, is very frail and has no strength in her hands or arms she also struggled to open and close her garden gate. Jill couldn't live independently without an assistance dog. Working with the charity's instructors, Astrid learnt to operate a system of pulleys and lines to open and close the heavy wooden gate, enabling Jill to get in and out of her garden with ease in her wheelchair. The pair were regular worshippers and concert goers at Salisbury Cathedral where Jill sells programmes before events. Other programme sellers were used to being left with nothing to do while a big crowd gathered around Jill to make a fuss of Astrid.

Astrid died in 2003 and Jill now shares her life with Yates, a black Labrador/retriever cross with boundless energy and a mind of his own. The couple are big fundraisers for Dogs for the Disabled but the task that Yates has made his own is to fetch the charger for Jill's electric wheelchair every evening. Without being told!

Annette also met Mark Drake and the faithful Hamish. 'Insecure, unsafe, stressed and nervous, with a fear of being trapped in a fire' was how Mark described his life before training with Hamish. Thanks to his dog Mark, who has been a wheelchair user since 1993, developed the confidence and ability to go shopping because he could call on Hamish to pick up what he needed from the shelf and take it to the counter and pay for it. Mark described Hamish as his best friend, partner and confidante and said he couldn't contemplate life without him.

Annette is already involved with a greyhound rescue charity and she was delighted to be able to help Dogs for the Disabled. Once again the appeal was a big success and raised in the region of £37,000.

Another client to hit the headlines with her dog was Norma Cail and her loyal little Finnish Lapphund, Tara, who won BBC Television's Community Champions award in 2001. Norma has chronic asthma and a serious heart condition. She has had several strokes that have debilitated the left side of her body, leaving her left leg paralysed and her hands and arms in splints. She is unable to stand and has been a full-time wheelchair user for twenty years. Despite her fragile health she is unendingly cheerful, never complains and is tireless in her efforts to raise awareness – and money – for Dogs for the Disabled.

Norma overcame her natural shyness and lack of confidence to become a registered speaker with the charity and gives an average of three fundraising talks a week. She always tells audiences how people in wheelchairs are ignored by others and never misses an opportunity to tell people about the difference her dog made to her life.

'When I used to fall out of my chair at home Tara would call the warden, then put a cushion under my head, grab the throw off the chair and put it over me. She saw the warden do it once so from then on she did it herself.'

At the start of Norma's talks, people would be entranced by Tara, a bright little dog with a gossamer-soft coat, but by the end of the talk they were also captivated by Norma, her courage and her warm personality.

Another important way of funding for the charity comes from corporate support and several companies provide valuable sponsorship.

Hill's Pet Nutrition has supported the charity since its early days by providing free food to puppies, dogs in training and qualified dogs. The company also sponsored Dogs for the Disabled staff uniforms.

Pet Protect provided free insurance for the first 150 dogs to qualify and substantially discounted premiums for all the others.

Snoozzzeee Dog Limited donated hundreds of luxurious dog duvets for the charity to sell, as well as helping with the cost of Outlook, the charity's magazine.

Ringpress Books Limited helped by sponsoring Outlook and supporting the charity in other ways.

Intervet UK Limited, produced vaccines used for puppies and dogs in training, and paid for the Creating Partnerships leaflet.

Missing Pets Bureau supported the charity with a cause-related marketing offer.

Pets at Home had a Charity of the Year relationship with Dogs for the Disabled for four years.

The Co-op Midlands supported the charity during 2006.

As the charity grew and became more widely known, it needed a figurehead to become its patron. The Marquess of Hertford, whose family home is Ragley Hall in Warwickshire, agreed to take on the role as well as becoming president of the Warwickshire Supporters' Group. Ragley Hall has been the family seat of the Conway Seymour family since Robert Hook built it in 1680. Set in 400 acres of parkland, woodland and gardens, it has breath-taking views of the Warwickshire countryside. The ninth Marquess of Hertford lives there with his Brazilian born wife Beatriz, four children, Gabriella, William, Edward and Antonia and the family's pet dogs.

The late Wendy Richard became vice-patron in 1996 after the first Lifeline appeal. Wendy was a dog lover and had a Cairn terrier called Miss Shirley Brahms, after the character she played in the 1970's TV comedy, Are You Being Served? Miss Shirley Brahms died in the summer of 2005. Wendy worked hard to support Dogs for the Disabled and made a point of visiting the charity's stands at Crufts and Discover Dogs whenever her hectic work schedule allowed. Wendy died from breast cancer in February 2009.

Dogs for the Disabled asked television presenter Anthea Turner to become its second vice-patron after the Liverpool Victoria Charity Snooker challenge in February 1998. Anthea was photographed with companies in Banbury who supported Dogs for the Disabled when the charity moved its headquarters to the town and she also visited its stand at Crufts. Anthea has two golden retrievers, Digger and Buddy, whose favourite pastime is to hunt out her most expensive shoes and play with them. Anthea says that at least with two dogs she loses the pair and not just one.

Peter Purves was invited to become Dogs for the Disabled's third vice-patron after he presented awards at the

Celebrating Partnerships event held at the Frances Hay Centre in September 2001. The first event of its kind, it acknowledged the success of the latest partnerships to train together. Peter presented the clients with certificates and gift bags, which were donated by Hill's Pet Nutrition. Peter has owned many dogs, including Newfoundlands, Pekinese and wire-haired dachshunds. Peter says he is delighted to support Dogs for the Disabled, especially as he has first-hand knowledge of what it is like to be disabled, albeit temporarily. A few years ago he fell 20 feet from the roof of his house when he was pruning some Virginia creeper and broke both his feet. The accident left him in a wheelchair for three and a half months. He now views life very differently.

Animal behaviourist Dr Roger Mugford became a vice-patron in 2002. After obtaining his BSc and PhD degrees at Hull University he went on to do post-doctoral research at the University of Pennsylvania, USA. After a spell at the Waltham (Pedigree) Centre for Pet Nutrition he founded the Animal Behaviour Centre, which specialises in the behaviour problems of domestic animals. Roger is a visiting lecturer at the Royal Veterinary College, London, and teaches his specialty to vets and students throughout the UK and overseas. As well as writing several books on animal behaviour and commentating on animal matters for television and radio, he finds time for a home life at his farm with his family and his menagerie of animals.

Brian Blessed is the most recent person to accept an invitation to become a vice-patron. Brian is probably best known for his acting roles in Flash Gordon, Star Wars and

Much Ado About Nothing but he also has a great sense of adventure and has climbed Mount Everest three times. Brian spent a day visiting the centre at Banbury and was able to see for himself how the dogs are trained to help disabled people.

'Everyone has their own Everest to climb and the work carried out by Dogs for the Disabled helps disabled people to achieve their dreams. I have always loved animals and I understand how these very special dogs can quite literally change lives and help a disabled person live life to the full,' he said.

Dogs for the Disabled needs funds more than ever before if it is to continue to support existing partnerships and to train more dogs to create new ones. Now that the charity has celebrated its twenty first anniversary there is a growing need for second and even third dogs. The average working life of an assistance dog is eight years. Some older clients will only need one dog but the younger ones will need several. It's not just a matter of one client one dog.

The charity places great emphasis on its relationships with a wide range of companies and is able to generate significant donations from this. Over the years, a more sophisticated mailing programme has been developed to keep the charity's donors in touch with Dogs for the Disabled's work. In addition, the charity is generating significant sums from charitable trusts – particularly as it develops new programmes of work.

However large or small the donation, every penny counts and is very much appreciated. For more information on ways to help or to make a donation please contact Dogs for the Disabled on 01295 252600. Alternatively, e-mail info@dogsforthedisabled.org or visit the web site: www.dogsforthedisabled.org

If you are a good-ideas person and one who likes to see the idea succeed, there is probably a supporters' group in your area that would like to hear from you. If you have a few hours to spare each month and would like to put them to good use, it's easy to get in touch via the above methods.

Chapter nine
What the future holds

Governance

Dogs for the Disabled was registered with the Charity Commission of England and Wales as a charitable trust in 1988 and since then has been governed by a board of trustees. In 2001 the trustees agreed that the charity should become incorporated as a charitable company, thereby giving the trustees limited liability status. Dogs for the Disabled became a charitable company in January 2003, when its registered charity number changed to 1092960. In 2007, the charity was registered in Scotland.

Developing New Services

Following the successful launch of the assistance dog training programme for children in 2005, Dogs for the Disabled has continued to research the many ways that dogs can assist disabled people.

When the charity started to work with children, it was surprised by the number of parents of children with autism who applied to have an assistance dog – 42% of the total applicants. The assistance dog training model used for children with physical disabilities is different from what is needed to train a dog to work with a child with autism.

However, responding to the demand from parents, Dogs for the Disabled established an autism assistance dog service in 2008.

For many years, staff at Dogs for the Disabled had been aware of other assistance dog programmes worldwide – most notably in Canada and Ireland – where children with autism are being trained successfully to work with a dog, resulting in significant benefits for the child and their family. This service is aimed at children between three and ten years of age, when the potential to modify behaviour is greatest.

The dog is trained to accompany the family into public places such as shopping centres and the positive impact of the dog is often quickly evident with the children clearly interacting with the environment and their family in ways that would have been impossible before. The adult is in control of the dog via a long lead while the child holds onto a harness attached to the dog and has a lead from the dog to their belt.

In the home the dog can help in a number of ways including breaking negative cycles of repetitive behaviour by nudging the child and distracting them. Repetitive behaviour can be very distressing for parents and sometimes even harmful to the child, so practical ways to modify such behaviour can be very valuable. Overall, parents are observing much calmer behaviour from their children and this has a knock-on effect to other siblings and the overall quality of family life.

New Facilities

When Dogs for the Disabled moved to the Frances Hay Centre in 2000 it was always planned to build a new kennel block and further client training facilities once the required money could be raised. New client training facilities and kennels were completed in July 2006. It was largely funded by donations from the staff and customers of the pet superstore chain Pets at Home and a personal donation from the founder of Pets at Home, Anthony Preston. Additional funding came from various charitable trusts. The facilities have proved to be a great asset to the charity and further kennels are planned for 2011.

The charity set up satellite centres in Weston Super Mare in Somerset in 2006 and at Nostell Priory in Yorkshire in 2008. These centres provide training facilities for clients and act as a base for several of the charity's instructors. In addition, the charity has a fundraiser based at Nostell, focusing on building community fundraising support in the area. The charity plans to develop these centres significantly over the next few years and has ambitious plans for further centres in the future, enabling clients to be supported and trained more locally.

The Wider Assistance Dog Movement

Since the first guide dog school was set up in Germany soon after the First World War, the international guide dog movement has grown substantially. The first hearing dog programme was started in the United States in the 1970s and programmes to assist people with other disabilities soon followed. Although the majority of programmes training assistance dogs are still based in the United States or in Europe, there has been a steady growth of programmes in other regions, most notably Australasia and Latin America.

Assistance Dogs International

Assistance Dogs International (ADI) is the worldwide umbrella body, set up in 1987, to support and promote the work of assistance dog programmes. ADI promotes standards of excellence in all areas of assistance dog acquisition, training and partnership, facilitates communication and learning among member organisations and educates the public as to benefits of assistance dogs and the work of ADI member programmes.

ADI changed its structure in 2007 and now has an international board and regional boards in North America and Europe. Further regions will soon be established in Asia, Australia, New Zealand and Latin America. Assistance Dogs Europe (ADEu) was set up in 2001 independently from ADI, but joined with ADI in 2007 as part of the restructuring.

ADI has over 180 member programmes worldwide and is run by a board of directors elected by the members. Membership is open to not-for-profit organisations that fulfil the application process. ADI sets standards for all aspects of assistance dog work worldwide and accredits programmes to ensure they are meeting these standards. In addition, it organises a series of regional and international networking events for members. The chief executive of Dogs for the Disabled, Peter Gorbing, was elected to the ADI board in

January 2002 and has been its President since 2007. Dogs
for the Disabled is proud of its leadership role in the
international movement and will continue to work closely
with other programmes across the world.

Assistance Dogs UK
Assistance Dogs UK was set up in the early 1990s with the
primary aim of improving access to places such as
supermarkets, restaurants, public transport and other public
facilities for people who depend on assistance dogs in the
UK.

Assistance dogs have public access rights under the
Disability Discrimination Act (1995) and it is unlawful for
disabled people to be discriminated against, or treated less
favourably, because of their disabilities. The Act requires
that service providers should make 'reasonable adjustment'
to their services and premises to enable disabled people
access and it is now well established that allowing people to
enter public places with their assistance dogs is a
'reasonable adjustment'.

The following charities are members of Assistance Dogs UK:
• Dogs for the Disabled
• The Guide Dogs for the Blind Association
• Hearing Dogs for Deaf People
• Canine Partners
• Support Dogs
• Dog Aid

Senior members of staff from these organisations meet together on a regular basis to ensure that access rights for their members are upheld and to look at ways of working together for mutual benefit.

Peter Gorbing,
Dogs for the Disabled
August 2009

Chapter ten
Skilled companion dogs

As every parent knows, there is nothing more painful than seeing your child suffer and being unable to do anything to help. As the mother of a twelve year old with cerebral palsy, Hilary Harris wondered what more she could do for her son, Tom.

Through a friend in Santa Rosa, California, Hilary was introduced to Jeannie Schulz, the widow of the Peanuts cartoonist Charles Schulz. Santa Rosa is home to Canine Companions for Independence, or CCI, the biggest assistance dog programme in the United States and Jeannie Schulz is its president. She arranged for Hilary to meet Corey Hudson, CCI's Executive Director, with a view to training a dog for Tom. Corey was unable to help but suggested Hilary contact Peter Gorbing at Dogs for the Disabled.

The charity had been thinking about training dogs for disabled children around the same time as Hilary contacted Peter and their subsequent conversation led to the launch of a children's pilot scheme, although Peter did explain to Hilary that, even if the charity went ahead with the idea, there was no guarantee they would find a suitable dog for Tom straight away.

Pets at Home provided financial support and the Skilled

Companion Dogs pilot scheme was launched in 2004. Three dogs with the necessary qualities to become skilled companions were selected for this special work and the charity held an information day to introduce disabled children and their families to them. This gave the instructors a chance to observe the reactions and behaviour of the children and dogs and also confirmed what everyone had suspected. The project was an important new field of work for the charity and proved to be extremely successful.

Tom Harris was one of the three children chosen to take part in the pilot scheme and he was partnered with Viggo. Teenager Kayleigh, who also has cerebral palsy, was partnered with Vicky and chocolate Labrador Yogi was partnered with twelve year old Daniel, who has Duchenne muscular dystrophy.

Skilled companion dogs are trained to help with four main areas of the child's development and Viggo, Vicky and Yogi led the way. They, and those that followed, were taught practical tasks, assistance with physiotherapy, development of life-skills and guided affection.

The early training for skilled companion dogs follows a similar course to that of the assistance dogs trained for adults. At the age of eight weeks the new recruits are placed with volunteer puppy socialisers for up to one year. They experience a wide variety of different sights and sounds and enjoy lots of encouragement and affection from their foster carers. By the time they are about twelve to fourteen months old and arrive at Dogs for the Disabled's training centre for their formal training, they are happy, fun loving dogs. The instructors and trainers use the tried and tested clicker and reward based training techniques: every time the dog responds correctly the trainer clicks and immediately gives a treat. Treats vary, according to the individual's dog's preference. Usually it is food but it could also be a toy, a cuddle or a game. The click and treat procedure is repeated over and over again, so the dog becomes proficient at the task in hand.

Recent research confirms that dogs can have a positive effect on children's development. Dogs for the Disabled trainers and instructors are experts in the field of specialist dog training and are convinced that dogs with special skills provide independence and therapeutic care to help disabled children with their future development.

Helen McCain is Director of Training and Development and co-ordinator of the children's project. She works with an instructor to guide the new partnerships through every aspect of the two-week residential training course at Banbury and to support them with regular visits when they return home. During the course the dog and child develop a special bond and become part of a team of three: child, carer and dog. The team learns the right commands to give the dog so it can help with practical tasks such as opening and closing doors, dressing or undressing the child, picking up named items such as a TV remote control, turning a light switch on or off or even pulling a duvet over the child at night.

Physiotherapy exercises can be painful and tedious and although they are necessary to help strengthen the body, children dislike them and often try to avoid doing them. All that changes once a Skilled Companion Dog comes on the scene. A dog needs regular grooming and the repetitive movement of this task can help strengthen the muscles in the hands and arms.

It wasn't long before Hilary Harris noticed that Tom was using his weaker left hand to stroke Viggo. Tom has difficulty using his left hand and before Viggo arrived he never volunteered to use it. Hilary says that since having Viggo, Tom actually wants to try and use both hands.

'That alone was a big step,' she said.

It is not always easy for children with disabilities to take active responsibility for their own care but an important part of the project is to encourage the children to take on responsibility for their dogs. They are encouraged to make sure their dog has the right amount of food, water exercise, grooming and health checks.

Kayleigh used to be very quietly spoken. But she has to give commands to Vicky and make herself understood. As a result, she can now project her voice much more effectively. Kayleigh feels that she's found a special friend.

'When I wake up in the morning I feel really excited and can't wait to get up. Vicky stands and watches me with her bright eyes and wagging tail, as if to say; "come on then, what adventures are we going to have today?".'

Disability often leads to feelings of isolation. Disabled children may not feel they have the same physical contact with friends and family that their peers do, but each Skilled Companion Dog is trained to cuddle on command. When

Tom, Kayleigh or Daniel feel like some much needed affection they just tell their canine friend 'paws up' and the cuddles commence. This warm, bodily contact goes a long way to counteract the children's feelings of loneliness.

Because of the severity of his condition Daniel can't just get up and go wherever and whenever he chooses. It affects and limits every aspect of his young life.

'I feel like I'm trapped in a box and I can't get out,' Daniel used to say. But in October 2004 Daniel started training with his new best friend, Yogi and gradually found he wasn't so trapped after all.

'I just love him. He puts his face up to mine and he wags his tail and makes me feel happy. He's so clever in the things that he does. Now I feel like I've always got a friend. I'm unsteady on my feet and I fall over easily. Yogi's been specially trained to bark so my mum will hear and come to help me any time of the day or night. That makes me feel safe and, for the first time in ages, I can do things by myself.

'If I can get dressed and undressed with Yogi's help it means that I don't have to ask my mum for everything. Yogi never says "in a minute Daniel" and he never tuts or frowns.'

Yogi has his bed in Daniel's room so he is there to attend to his needs or take a note to Mary if Daniel needs human assistance. The first thing that greets him in the morning is a wagging tail, and that means Daniel wakes up with a smile.

Mary, his mother, explains. 'Daniel wasn't like his older brother as a baby and parts of his development didn't seem right. He would sleep all the time and wouldn't sit up like a normal baby. As he grew older he did learn to walk but just couldn't manage stairs or to push himself up from a sitting position.

'After Daniel was diagnosed with Duchenne Muscular Dystrophy I just felt crushed and I went around in a daze for two weeks.

'It was just too horrible to contemplate that my son was going to be disabled and his life was going to be so limited. Worse still, I can't protect him from what he has to go through.

'Having a child with a disability has an effect on the whole family. Sometimes I need to do more for him than for his brother and sister and that can be extremely hard for them to understand.'

Despite this, Mary is still as determined to help Daniel as she was the day she found out about his condition.

'I spend hours on the internet looking for services that may be available to him. That's how I found out about Dogs for the Disabled and the new UK project to help disabled children.'

Soon after Mary contacted the charity, the family was invited to go along to the information day in Banbury.

'I remember when they brought Yogi in,' says Daniel. 'This handsome dog just came up to me and wagged his tail and snuffled his nose into my hands. He was just brilliant. I hoped that I'd get a dog just like Yogi.'

Neither Mary nor Daniel could believe it when they got the call to say they'd been accepted onto the pilot scheme and the dog the instructors had in mind for Daniel was Yogi.

With the help of the instructor and hard work from Daniel, Mary and Yogi they formed a team very quickly. Yogi's magic began to work.

When you walk down the street with a child in a wheelchair people don't usually know where to look or how to react but since Yogi has been accompanying the family on shopping trips all that has changed. People stop and smile. They want to talk to Daniel and find out more about Yogi, resulting in a boost to Daniel's confidence and making him feel more accepted.

Yogi might be the newest member of the household but he has changed the whole family's life in such a positive way. This was never more true than when Daniel and Yogi were short listed for the 'Friends for Life' award at Crufts Dog Show in 2006.

Six dogs were nominated for showing acts of bravery, companionship or help in some way. A short film was made of each nominee and shown several times over the four days of the world's biggest dog show, and members of the public were invited to vote for their favourite partnership.

Daniel and his family travelled to Birmingham from Newcastle and were mobbed when they reached the Dogs for the Disabled stand – people said they were so touched and impressed by their partnership. Everyone who visited the stand said they had voted for them.

On the final evening, just before the judging for Best in Show, the Friends for Life nominees entered the main ring and waited nervously for the results. Daniel bravely entered the ring alone. His family watched anxiously from the sidelines.

Finally the winner was announced. It was Daniel and Yogi by a mile. More than 150,000 votes were cast over the four days of Crufts. Daniel and Yogi received 145,000 of them and when they received their award they also got a standing ovation from the crowd, most of whom were moved to tears. Thanks to Yogi, Daniel has a new best friend, his mum has someone to make her smile and his bother and sister have a new rough and tumble play-mate.

Epilogue
Moving on – Sarah and Demi

On 3rd October 2002 Jade walked out of my life and left me devastated, with tears in my eyes, a lump in my throat and a broken heart. Jade, my little ray of sunshine, my inspiration for this book, the one who walked into my life four and a half years previously and put a smile back on my face had been retired. The old feelings of emptiness, isolation and lack of confidence came flooding back instantly, just as they had done before I had an assistance dog and after Zach left.

My smile also diminished for a time, like a light going out. My reason for getting up in the morning had gone. It was a struggle to keep going and the physical pain became worse because I found myself having to do the jobs Jade once did so efficiently and so willingly.

In July 2002, following an aftercare visit to Coventry, my instructor and I agreed to semi-retire Jade with immediate effect. This was because of her heightened sensitivity to traffic noise and her refusal to work in town. I continued to work her around home and local shops, but the situation became difficult for both of us as she missed her long walks with me and I had to leave her behind whenever I went into town or visited an area where there was heavy traffic.

Sensitive and intelligent as she was, she became increasingly confused with her semi-retired status so, for both our sakes, Jade went to a foster home until a suitable permanent home was found. As long as she had human contact, toys, country walks and fields where she could be free to let off steam, I knew she would enjoy full retirement.

We'd been through so much together it was difficult to let go and I have so many memories of her. She loved to chase birds and squirrels in the park, following her natural herding instincts I suppose, and I used to watch them disappear into the trees. Jade would have a puzzled expression on her face – you could almost hear her thinking 'they're not supposed to do that'. Then she'd sit and bark furiously at the branches, willing the squirrels to come down and give her a game of chase. She never quite grasped the fact that the squirrel went up there to hide from her in the first place.

Chasing squirrels nearly led to tragedy one day. Jade caught sight of one disappearing into the undergrowth and went in after it, ignoring my pleas for her to return to me. The next minute I heard a yelp and my blood ran cold. Eventually she limped, whimpering, out of the bushes and rolled over to reveal a gaping wound on her underside. An operation and an overnight stay at the vet's followed. The gash had just missed a main artery. A few millimetres nearer and Jade would have died. Fortunately, with a lot of professional expertise and my nursing skills, she made a full recovery. But she couldn't work for two months and it was during this time I realised just how much she did for me on a daily basis. The cause of the injury? A dumped television. Jade is living proof that dumping rubbish can be dangerous.

This poem was sent to me by the author Jillie Wheeler to celebrate Dogs for the Disabled's 150th partnership. It sums up exactly what Jade meant to me.

JADE

You're one in a million,
You're special to me,
Affectionate, loyal
And good company.
You're there when I'm lonely
And life seems a bore,
You cheer me and offer
A comforting paw.
The look in your eyes
Says you quite understand,
As you thrust a be-whiskered
Wet nose in my hand.
You never desert me
Wherever I go,
You're a far better friend
Than some people I know!
I thank you by writing
This short monologue,
To my faithful, devoted
Companion – my dog

© Jillie Wheeler 1979

Jade died peacefully in her sleep on January 19th 2009 aged 13.

In October 2004 I got the call I had been waiting for and my next assistance dog arrived in the form of a black Labrador x golden retriever called Demi. A laid-back and affectionate soul who takes everything in her stride, she has a gentle but persuasive nature and likes nothing better than to walk round with a soft toy in her mouth or for use as a chin rest when she goes to bed.

Demi settled in well to family life. Sidney the cat soon showed her who was boss on their first meeting by swiping her across the nose. Demi retreated under the table and took some persuading to come out. Our instructor placed a glove on the floor for Demi to fetch but with Sidney still in the room she wasn't going to move. The glove was replaced with a tasty dog treat which we felt sure would encourage her out of her hiding place, but quick as a flash Sidney turned round and ate the treat. However a couple of days later the pair of them were sitting side by side in the garden. They are now very close, often sharing Demi's bed and when it is time for a walk Sidney comes too.

Demi and I have also grown together in confidence and enjoy a very special bond. As all dog owners know, every dog has its own special place in your heart. Jade had hers. And now Demi has hers too.

Author's note

It has been a pleasure and privilege working on this book with Sarah Carr, whom I met when I was working as press officer for Dogs for the Disabled. During my time with the charity I met many clients and learned at first hand what an enormous difference their marvellous assistance dogs made to their lives. I am grateful to all of them for allowing us to tell their stories. Sadly, time does not stand still and over the past few years some of the people whose stories appear on these pages have died. So too have some of the dogs. But their stories live on in the hearts and minds of their friends, families and colleagues. This book, the story of Dogs for the Disabled, is our tribute to them.

Jackie Williamson
July 2009.

Further reading

If you would like to teach your dog how to carry out simple tasks, a new book by dog behaviourist Gwen Bailey is full of practical advice. *Clever Dog* is published by Collins and costs £10.99. Gwen's next book, *'How to Train a Superdog'* has more about how to train dogs in a positive way, how to understand them and insights into how they think. For more information visit Gwen's website: www.dogbehaviour.com

About the writers

Sarah Carr was born in Royal Leamington Spa in 1962 and lived there until the age of 11 when the family moved to the Isle of Arran in Scotland. Sarah left school at 17 to work in the local Tourist Information Centre. Later she travelled south to London to work as a hotel receptionist and as a typist in a French bank. While in London she met and married her husband Martin, who has constantly supported her. The couple moved to Warwick in 1993 and Sarah has been involved with the charity Dogs for the Disabled since 1994. Her assistance dog, Jade, inspired her to write this book. Because of the strong bond that they shared, Sarah wanted others to know what a difference having an assistance dog makes to a disabled person's life.

Jackie Williamson is an author, journalist, poet, editor and publisher. She lives close to the sea in west Wales with her husband and two beagles. Publishing credits include:
Writing Letters and Reports for Thames Valley Police (textbook) 1996
Banbury (anthology) Published by Ottakars 2001
In Her Element (anthology) Published by Honno 2007
Cevamp, Mike and Me Published by Acorns Publishing 2007
Memory Seeds (poetry) Published by Acorns Publishing 2009
Coming soon: Whale Steak and Chips – an elderly widow reflects on her childhood, teen years, married life and old age.